3RD **Edition**

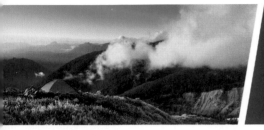

# WASHINGTON

## YOUR CAR-CAMPING GUIDE TO SCENIC BEAUTY, THE SOUNDS OF NATURE, AND AN ESCAPE FROM CIVILIZATION

**Best Tent Camping: Washington**
Copyright © 2019 by Michelle L. Kozlowski
Copyright © 2005 and 2009 by Jeanne Louise Pyle
Printed in the United States of America
Published by Menasha Ridge Press
Distributed by Publishers Group West
Third edition, first printing

**Library of Congress Cataloging-in-Publication Data is on file with the Library of Congress**
ISBN 978-0-89732-681-0; eISBN 978-0-89732-682-7

Cover design by Scott McGrew
Cover photos by Ellie Kozlowski and scnhnc052008/Shutterstock (top)
Text design by Jonathan Norberg
Photos by Ellie Kozlowski, except where noted on page
Project editor: Kate Johnson
Copyeditor: Dianna Stirpe
Proofreader: Laura Franck
Indexer: Rich Carlson

*Cover photo:* Panorama Point Campground (see page 94) and a campsite in the Washington Cascades (top)

## MENASHA RIDGE PRESS
An imprint of AdventureKEEN
2204 First Ave. S, Ste. 102
Birmingham, AL 35233
800-443-7227, fax 205-326-1012

Visit menasharidge.com for a complete listing of our books and for ordering information. Contact us at our website, at facebook.com/menasharidge, or at twitter.com/menasharidge with questions or comments. To find out more about who we are and what we're doing, visit blog.menasharidge.com.

3RD Edition

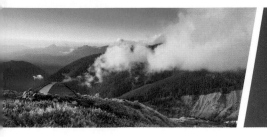

# BEST ⛺ TENT
# Camping

# WASHINGTON

## YOUR CAR-CAMPING GUIDE TO SCENIC BEAUTY, THE SOUNDS OF NATURE, AND AN ESCAPE FROM CIVILIZATION

## Ellie Kozlowski

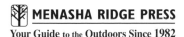

**MENASHA RIDGE PRESS**
Your Guide to the Outdoors Since 1982

# Washington Campground Locator Map

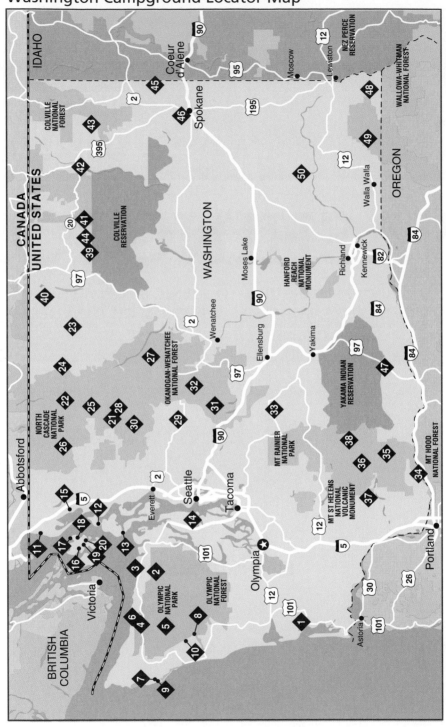

# CONTENTS

# Map Legend

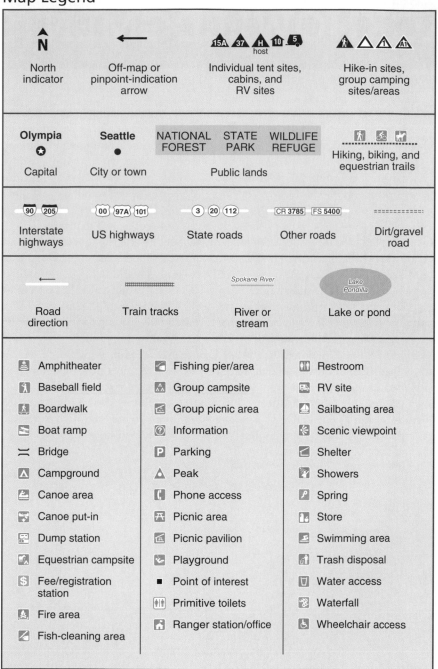

**N** — North indicator

← — Off-map or pinpoint-indication arrow

15A 37 H 10 5 host — Individual tent sites, cabins, and RV sites

— Hike-in sites, group camping sites/areas

**Olympia** ✪ — Capital

**Seattle** ● — City or town

NATIONAL FOREST   STATE PARK   WILDLIFE REFUGE — Public lands

— Hiking, biking, and equestrian trails

90 205 — Interstate highways

00 97A 101 — US highways

3 20 112 — State roads

CR 3785   FS 5400 — Other roads

— Dirt/gravel road

← — Road direction

— Train tracks

*Spokane River* — River or stream

*Lake Pondilla* — Lake or pond

Amphitheater

Baseball field

Boardwalk

Boat ramp

Bridge

Campground

Canoe area

Canoe put-in

Dump station

Equestrian campsite

Fee/registration station

Fire area

Fish-cleaning area

Fishing pier/area

Group campsite

Group picnic area

Information

Parking

Peak

Phone access

Picnic area

Picnic pavilion

Playground

■ Point of interest

Primitive toilets

Ranger station/office

Restroom

RV site

Sailboating area

Scenic viewpoint

Shelter

Showers

Spring

Store

Swimming area

Trash disposal

Water access

Waterfall

Wheelchair access

# ACKNOWLEDGMENTS

**Without the encouragement and support** I received from my community of friends, writers, yogis, outdoorspeople, and family, I would not have been able to visit so many campgrounds in so short a time. Thank you to Tim Jackson and Brett Ortler of AdventureKEEN for placing this project with me and setting me up for an incredible year of exploring Washington State. Thank you to everyone else at AdventureKEEN who touched this manuscript, including the cartographers, who turned my "drawings" into beautiful campground maps, and the marketing team, proofreader, fact checkers, and editors. Special shout out to my project editor Kate Johnson—thank you for helping push this project through to print.

My heart is full of gratitude for all of my camping buddies and explorers extraordinaire: Rachel Toor, Lisa Laughlin, Maya Jewell Zeller, Laura Read, Jill Leininger, Sean Koenig, and Denise Miller—it was an absolute pleasure (and a heck of a good time) to do research with each of you. Thank you to Esther Whitmore for helping me modify my vehicle to fit even more supplies (including a platform bed if I needed it). Thank you to all of you who offered advice and revealed your favorite campgrounds (rather than keeping them a secret). Your recommendations proved invaluable.

I would be remiss if I didn't thank the late Jeanne Pyle for pioneering this series. I had a blast tracing her routes across the state and reevaluating the sites she deemed worthy of inclusion in this book. Her original research was helpful beyond measure.

And a giant thank-you to my partner and greatest supporter, Jonah Kozlowski, who is always ready to chuck a tent in the car and drive for hours down roads of varying conditions toward any adventure that involves a campfire (or the potential to see a bear).

—Ellie Kozlowski

# PREFACE

In our fast-paced technological world of screens and notifications, many of us are still drawn to the pleasures of getting out into the woods and sitting around a campfire. Is it the simplicity? Is it the smell of a marshmallow roasting? The sound of a river rolling by? Could it be the near-complete lack of cell service? It's hard to put your finger on it, but I like to think it's the pace. Slowing down feels really, really good. Once I find myself in the habit of taking a break from it all, I only want to take more breaks, by which I mean I want to plan more camping trips. I've ventured to the far corners of beautiful Washington State to bring you what I've determined are the best campgrounds for a peaceful getaway. I tend to favor fewer frills in exchange for a more secluded feel, farther from major thoroughfares. Even so, I've included campgrounds with luxe amenities close to cities as well. I truly adore each campground included here.

If you're a novice camper or new to Washington, you will learn a lot in these pages. And if you're an experienced outdoorsperson and find yourself stuck in the groove of visiting only your favorite three spots, I have 50 solid recommendations for you.

I hope you take every opportunity to enjoy this newly updated and expanded edition of *Best Tent Camping: Washington.* So far, the natural disasters have failed to hinder my best attempts to bring you the most current news from the camping scene (but always check online or call the ranger station for weather and road conditions!), and I refuse to be held personally responsible for what effect Mount St. Helens might have on the state of things. Or the big earthquake. Enjoy these spots while you can.

Happy camping,

—Ellie Kozlowski

# BEST CAMPGROUNDS

# BEST FOR QUIET

# BEST FOR SECURITY

# BEST FOR BEAUTY

# BEST FOR CLEANLINESS

View from the bluff at Dungeness Recreation Area (see page 22)

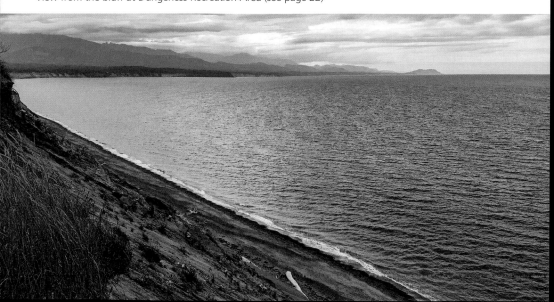

# BEST FOR FISHING

# BEST FOR HORSE TRAILS

# BEST FOR SWIMMING

## BEST FOR HIKING

## BEST FOR PADDLING

## BEST FOR PADDLING *(continued)*

## BEST FOR BOATING

## BEST FOR WATERFALLS

## BEST FOR FAMILIES

## BEST FOR BIRDING

## BEST FOR BICYCLING

## BEST FOR WILDLIFE VIEWING

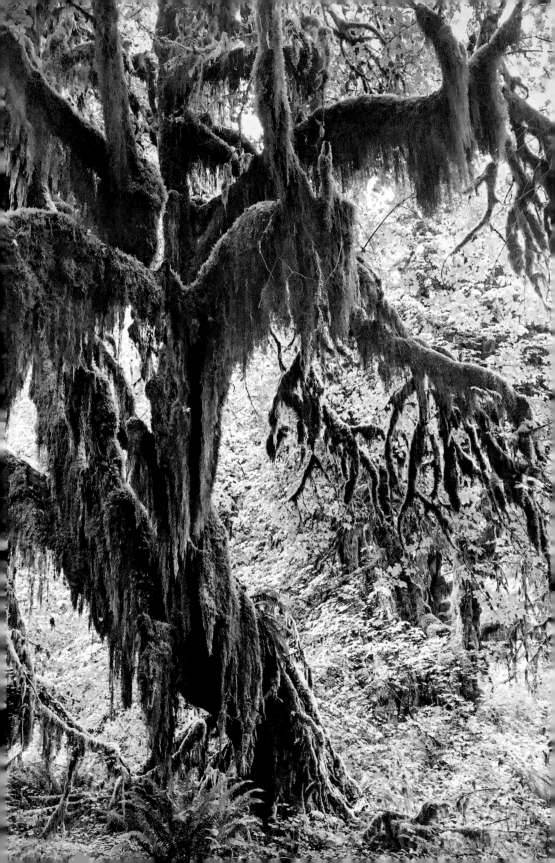

# INTRODUCTION

## A WORD ABOUT THIS BOOK AND WASHINGTON TENT CAMPING

*From wide, sandy beaches to volatile,* snowcapped volcanoes to narrow river gorges, Washington rivals its neighbor Oregon as a place of different but equally unparalleled natural beauty and diversity. As with Oregon, extremes of climate, terrain, and vegetation can be experienced in just a single day's outing. The campgrounds included in this book are representative of the variety that makes Washington a beloved destination for those who seek outstanding outdoor adventures, either for a quick weekend getaway or an extended tour.

And for those who seek that adventure farther afield than most and who value an experience that's long on solitude, serenity, and space, be aware that you may have to drive farther and climb higher and plan more creatively. Although Washington ranks among the top five states in designated wilderness acreage, that acreage still constitutes only about 10% of the state's total land. With more and more people flocking to the scenic natural splendors beyond city limits, this pushes the capacity for a true wilderness experience to new boundaries.

Encountering RVs in the most unlikely of places, one has to wonder if it isn't more comforting to think of wilderness as a state of mind rather than an actual place. I have observed that for some tent campers, it's satisfaction enough just to pitch a tent alongside several hundred others in midsummer at a busy nearby state park. For others, simply being able to drive to a campground immediately eliminates it from consideration. If your sentiment lies somewhere between these two extremes, you should find the offerings in this book appealing.

A trend I have noticed in the past few years is a bit of a "good news, bad news" report, but I prefer to look at it as an encouraging sign. In the larger, more developed campgrounds run by the various agencies that have a hand in developing, managing, and maintaining the public lands of Washington, it's now not uncommon to find a loop of sites designated as "tent camping" and another defined as "RVs/trailers." The tent-camping sites are more rustic, without electric hookups, and usually with better vegetation between sites. The bad news is that they often get taken by the overflow of rigs and trailers that get there before the tent campers (certainly not because they're faster) and squeeze themselves into the parking space. One problem solved; another one created. Still, it's good to see that there is sensitivity to two very different styles of camping within the same compound.

Naturally, there are factors besides crowds that affect every camping trip, from a last-minute urge to slip out of town to a backcountry expedition planned months in advance. Here's some information that will prove useful whether you're a first-time camper in Washington or a veteran who can always use a few reminders.

**OPPOSITE:** Hall of Mosses Trail, Hoh Rain Forest (page 28)

## WEST VERSUS EAST

For a traveler new to the state, the most distinctive feature in Washington is the difference in climate, terrain, and, to some degree, lifestyle between its western and eastern regions. While this book groups the campgrounds in fairly broad geographical regions simply for locator purposes, west and east here are, by and large, defined by the Pacific Crest National Scenic Trail, or simply the Pacific Crest Trail (PCT), which you'll find on most of the topo and Forest Service maps. The PCT begins at the United States–Canada border and follows the spine of the Cascade Range down through Washington and Oregon, continuing on into California to its end at the Mexican border. In Washington, it starts on the western edge of Pasayten Wilderness and plunges due south into fearsome terrain that can make even the most intrepid mountain goat question the sanity of its lifestyle. The trail exits the state into Oregon a tad more sedately just a few miles east of Beacon Rock State Park (page 120), crossing the Columbia River over the Bridge of the Gods.

## CASCADIA MARINE TRAIL

Since its creation in 1993, the Cascadia Marine Trail has grown to include more than 160 day-use sites and 65 campgrounds, some of which are highlighted here. The water trail is on Puget Sound and offers 150 miles' worth of paddling from Olympia to Point Roberts (at the Canada–US border). It earned a designation from the White House as one of only 16 National Millennium Trails. Several campgrounds reserve a site specifically for boat-in folks traveling on the marine trail.

## THE RATINGS AND RATING CATEGORIES

Within the scope of the original campground criteria for this book—accessible by car and preferably not by RV, scenic, and as close to a wilderness setting as possible—each campground has its own characteristics. The best way to deal with these varying attributes was to devise a rating system that highlights each campground's best features. On our five-star ranking system, five is the highest rating and one is the lowest. So if you're looking for a campground that is beautiful and achingly quiet, look for five stars in both of those categories. If you're more interested in a campground that has excellent security and cavernous campsites, look for five stars in the spaciousness and security categories. Keep in mind that these ratings are based somewhat on the subjective views of the author and her sources.

★★★★★     The site is **ideal** in that category.

★★★★     The site is **exemplary** in that category.

★★★     The site is **very good** in that category.

★★     The site is **above average** in that category.

★     The site is **acceptable** in that category.

## BEAUTY

If this category needs any explanation, it's simply to say that the true beauty of a campground is not always what you can see but what you can't see. Or hear. Like a freeway. Or roaring motorboats. Or the *crack, pop, pop, boom* of a rifle range. An equally important factor for me on the beauty scale is the condition of the campground itself and to what extent it has been left in its natural state. Beauty also, of course, takes into consideration any fabulous views of mountains, water, or other natural phenomena.

## PRIVACY

No one who enjoys the simplicity of tent camping wants to be walled in on all sides by RVs the size of tractor trailers. This category goes hand in hand with the previous one because part of the beauty of a campsite has to do with the privacy of its surroundings. If you've ever crawled out of your tent to embrace a stunning summer morning in your skivvies and found several pairs of very curious eyes staring at you from the neighbor's picture window, you know what I mean. I look for campsites that are graciously spaced with lots of heavy foliage in between. You usually have to drive a little deeper into the campground complex for these sites.

## SPACIOUSNESS

This is the category you toss the coin on and keep your fingers crossed. I'm not as much of a stickler for this category because I'm happy if there's room to park the car off the main campground road, enough space to pitch a two- or four-person tent in a reasonably flat and dry spot, a picnic table for meal preparation, and a fire pit safely away from the tenting area. At most campgrounds, site spaciousness is sacrificed for site privacy and vice versa. Sometimes you get extremely lucky and have both. Don't be greedy.

## QUIET

Again, this category goes along with the beauty of a place. When I go camping, I want to hear the sounds of nature. You know, birds chirping, the wind sighing, a surf crashing, a brook babbling. Call me crazy, but it's not always possible to control the noise volume of your fellow campers, so the closer you can get to natural sounds that can drown them out, the better. Actually, when you have a chance to listen to the quiet of nature, you'll find that it's really rather noisy. But what a lovely cacophony!

## SECURITY

Quite a few of the campgrounds in this book are in remote and primitive places without on-site security patrol. In essence, you're on your own. Common sense is a great asset in these cases. Don't leave expensive gear or valuable camera equipment lying around your campsite or even within view inside your car. If you're at a hosted site, you may feel more comfortable leaving any valuables with the host (if they're willing). Or let them know if you'll be gone for an extended period of time so they can keep an eye on your things.

Unfortunately, even in lightly camped areas, vandalism is a common camping problem. In many places, the wild animals can do as much damage as a human being. If you leave food inside your tent or around the campsite, don't be surprised if things look slightly ransacked when you return. The most frequent visitors to food-strewn campsites are birds, squirrels, chipmunks, deer, and bears.

## CLEANLINESS

By and large, all the campgrounds in this book should rank five stars for this category. Park- and forest-service personnel work hard to keep campgrounds clean and free of litter and unnecessary debris. The only time they tend to fall a bit short of expectation is on busy summer weekends. This is usually only in the larger, more developed compounds. In more remote areas, the level of cleanliness is most often dependent on the good habits of the campers themselves. Keep that in mind wherever you camp. If the sign says PACK IT IN, PACK IT OUT, do as you're told. You can dump your garbage at the first gas fill-up spot. Don't expect someone to pick up after you at the campsite.

## THE CAMPGROUND PROFILE

The campground profile is where you'll find the nitty-gritty details. Not only is the property described, but also readers can get a general idea of the recreational opportunities available—what's in the area and perhaps suggestions for touristy activities.

## THE CAMPGROUND LOCATOR MAP AND MAP LEGEND

Use the campground locator map on page iv to pinpoint the location of each campground. Each campground's number follows it throughout this guidebook: from that campground locator map, to the table of contents, and to the profile's first page. A map legend that details the symbols found on the campground-layout maps appears on page vii.

## CAMPGROUND-LAYOUT MAPS

Each profile contains a detailed map of campground sites, internal roads, facilities, and other key items.

## CAMPGROUND ENTRANCE GPS COORDINATES

All 50 profiles in this guidebook include the GPS coordinates for each campground. The intersection of the latitude (north) and longitude (west) coordinates orient you at the entrance. Please note that this guidebook uses the degree–decimal minute format for presenting the GPS coordinates. Example:

**N46° 41.017' W123° 53.265'**

To convert GPS coordinates from degrees, minutes, and seconds to the above degree–decimal minute format, divide the seconds by 60. For more on GPS technology, visit usgs.gov.

# WEATHER

Prevailing conditions year-round in western Washington (with one exception) are mild and damp. Not so much rain, actually, as a healthy supply of gray clouds and mist. The exception is a phenomenon known as the banana belt, which is an area with drier weather from Sequim on the Olympic Peninsula across the Strait of Juan de Fuca, into the San Juan Islands, catching the western edge of Whidbey Island and Anacortes, and continuing northeast over parts of Whatcom County. Late summer and early fall are the most dependable for a lovely string of dry, sunny, warm days just about anywhere in western Washington.

In eastern Washington, conditions are prairielike at lower elevations, and in the summer, the heat is on—searingly hot and dust-bowl dry. You'll want to head for the hills, which won't be all that noticeably cooler by day but can get chilly at night. Severe thunderstorms can be the biggest threat to outdoor activity, and this, in turn, can spark instantaneous wildfires and flash floods. At higher elevations on both western and eastern mountain slopes, snow is not uncommon even in midsummer. Sudden changes in weather conditions are always a consideration, so pack for the weather and whatever activities you may be planning.

## ROAD CONDITIONS

Many of the campgrounds in this book are reached by minimally maintained access roads. Since we were looking for spots that are somewhat off the beaten path (and away from the routes those dreaded RVs travel), access roads can be rougher than you might expect. Check current road conditions before venturing too far if you are unsure of what you may encounter. And be sure that you have a good current road atlas or U.S. Forest Service map with you. The maps in this book are designed to help orient you, nothing more. Although we've provided directions at the end of each entry, you'll find it useful to have more detailed maps with you when traveling around most of these campgrounds. I also download an offline map of each area I plan to visit before I hit the road. Local and district offices that oversee the management of most of these campgrounds are the best source for detailed paper maps (see Appendix B, page 179, for more information on these agencies).

## RESTRICTIONS

More people using an area usually means more restrictions. State and federal agencies manage most of the campgrounds in this book. Check with the proper authorities for current regulations on recreational activities, such as permits for day-use parking, backcountry travel, licenses for hunting and fishing, mountain bikes in designated areas, and so on. We've included some restrictions in the Key Information sections of each campground description, but because restrictions can change, you still need to check before you go. Be aware that many national-forest and state-park parking areas now require day-use fees or annual passes. Passes can be purchased at any Forest Service office, ranger station, or park office, as well as at numerous campgrounds and outdoor-retailer outlets.

## FIRES

Campfire regulations are subject to seasonal conditions. Usually there are signs posted at campgrounds or ranger district offices. Please be sure you're aware of the current situation, and never make a campfire anywhere other than in existing fire pits at developed sites. Never, ever toss a match or cigarette idly in the brush or alongside the road. It's not only a littering consideration; a single match can be the destruction of that beautiful forest you were just admiring.

## WATER

Many of the campgrounds in this book are remote enough that potable water is not available. No matter how remote you may think you are, don't risk drinking straight from mountain streams, creeks, or lakes. Washington strives to keep its natural waters pure, but it's not immune to that nasty parasite called *Giardia lamblia,* which causes horrific stomach cramps and long-term diarrhea. If you don't have drinking water or purification tablets with you, bring any untreated water to a rolling boil for 1 minute—3 minutes if you're at an altitude over 6,562 feet. This will seem like a hassle if you're dry as a bone at the end of a long day of activity, but believe me, it's worth the few minutes of waiting for the agony you will avoid.

## FIRST AID KIT

A useful first aid kit may contain more items than you might think necessary. These are just the basics. Prepackaged kits in waterproof bags are available. As a preventive measure, always take along sunscreen and insect repellent. Even though quite a few items are listed here, they pack down into a small space:

- Adhesive bandages
- Antibiotic ointment
- Antiseptic or disinfectant, such as Betadine or hydrogen peroxide
- Benadryl or the generic equivalent, diphenhydramine (in case of allergic reactions)
- Butterfly-closure bandages
- Elastic bandages or joint wraps
- Emergency poncho
- Epinephrine in a prefilled syringe (for severe allergic reactions to bee stings, etc.)
- Gauze (one roll and six 4-by-4-inch pads)
- Ibuprofen or acetaminophen
- Insect repellent
- LED flashlight or headlamp
- Matches or pocket lighter
- Mirror for signaling passing aircraft
- Moleskin/Spenco 2nd Skin
- Pocketknife or multipurpose tool
- Sunscreen, lip balm
- Waterproof first aid tape
- Whistle (it's more effective in signaling rescuers than your voice)

# FLORA AND FAUNA PRECAUTIONS

## POISONOUS PLANTS

Recognizing poison ivy, oak, and sumac and avoiding contact with them are the most effective ways to prevent the painful, itchy rashes associated with these plants. Poison ivy ranges from a thick, tree-hugging vine to a shaded ground cover, 3 leaflets to a leaf; poison oak occurs as either a vine or shrub, with 3 leaflets as well; and poison sumac flourishes in swampland, each leaf containing 7–13 leaflets. Urushiol, the oil in the sap of these plants, is responsible for the rash. Usually within 12–14 hours of exposure (but sometimes later), raised lines and/or blisters will appear, accompanied by a terrible itch. Refrain from scratching because bacteria under fingernails can cause infection. Wash and dry the rash thoroughly, applying a calamine lotion or other product to help dry out the rash. If itching or blistering is severe, seek medical attention. Remember that oil-contaminated clothes, pets, or hiking gear can easily cause an irritating rash on you or someone else, so wash not only any exposed parts of your body but also anything else that might have come into contact with the oil.

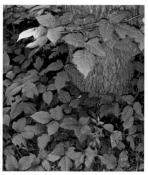
Poison ivy

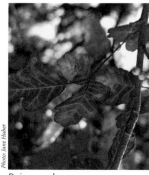
Poison oak

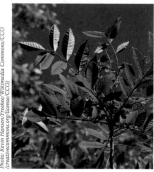
Poison sumac

## MOSQUITOES

Mosquitoes are common, especially on the east side of the state, especially in early summer. Skeeters, along with no-see-ums, can plague coastal areas. Likewise, deer and horse flies are active during the day near streams, ponds, lakes, and marshy areas. Their sharp bites are painful and can itch for days; avoid scratching so as not to cause infection. Though it's very rare, especially in Washington, individuals can become infected with the West Nile virus by being bitten by an infected mosquito. Culex mosquitoes, the primary varieties that can transmit West Nile to humans, thrive in urban rather than natural areas. They lay their eggs in stagnant water and can breed in any standing water that remains for more than five days. Most people infected with the West Nile virus have no symptoms of illness, but some may become ill, usually 3–15 days after being bitten.

Anytime you expect mosquitoes to be buzzing around, you may want to wear protective clothing, such as long sleeves, long pants, and socks. Loose-fitting, light-colored clothing is best. Spray clothing with insect repellent. Remember to follow the instructions on the repellent and to take extra care to protect children against these insects. You may want to treat your clothing with permethrin before heading to a particularly mosquito-filled area.

## SNAKES

We only have one venomous snake in Washington: the Western rattlesnake. Despite their name, they only live on the east side of the state. Hibernation season is typically October–April. The rest of the year you might see them in the desert, basking in the sun on the trail or hiding under a rock or log. They can be anywhere from 18 inches to 4 feet in length, have a wide triangular head, facial pits, large dark spots or diamonds, and a rattle at the end of their tail. Rattlesnakes won't bite unless threatened. If you see one, do not approach it or leap over it; the best rule is to leave the way you came or give a wide berth as you hike past, making sure any hiking companions (including dogs) do the same. If you get bit, seek medical attention.

When hiking, stick to well-used trails, and wear over-the-ankle boots and loose-fitting long pants. Do not step or put your hands beyond your range of detailed visibility, and avoid wandering around in the dark. Step *onto* logs and rocks, never *over* them, and be especially careful when climbing rocks. Always avoid walking through dense brush or willow thickets. The snakes you will most likely see while hiking will be nonvenomous species and subspecies.

## TICKS

Ticks are often found on brush and tall grass, where they seem to be waiting to hitch a ride on a warm-blooded passerby. Adult ticks can appear anytime from January to May and again in October and November. The black-legged tick, commonly called the deer tick, is the primary carrier of Lyme disease. Lyme disease is rare in Washington (about 0–3 cases are reported per year). We can thank the soft tick *Ornithodoros hermsi* (common in rural mountainous areas of eastern Washington) for tick-borne relapsing fever (0-12 cases per year) and the American dog tick and Rocky Mountain wood tick for Rocky Mountain spotted fever (0-2 cases per year). These ticks exist across the state and tend to hang out in wooded regions, medium-height grasses, shrubs in wetlands, or forest meadows. Wear light-colored clothing to make it easier for you to spot ticks before they migrate to your skin. At the end of the hike, visually check hair, back of neck, armpits, and socks. During your post-hike shower, take a moment to do a more complete body check. For ticks that are already embedded, removal with tweezers is best. Grasp the tick close to your skin, and remove it by pulling straight out firmly. Do your best to remove the head, but do not twist. Use disinfectant solution on the wound.

## COUGARS AND WOLVES

You've probably never seen a cougar, but you've likely been seen by one if you've spent time hiking in Washington, western or eastern. That's what they say, anyway. Campgrounds will often have an information placard about cougars if they're likely to inhabit the surrounding area. Cougar attacks are highly unlikely.

You likely won't see a pack of wolves hanging out either, but you never know what you'll come across in the Okanogan or northeast part of the state. They are protected and endangered in Washington. They are even less likely to be spotted than cougars and are usually in deep wilderness areas.

Hike in groups, and don't be afraid to make noise and talk. It's best to make predators aware of your presence. If you do encounter a cougar or wolf, stop and stand tall. Make yourself look even larger—raise your arms overhead, lift your jacket up. Pick up children and pets, and never run, turn your back, crouch, or hide. Cougars and wolves instinctively want to chase, so don't make any sudden movements. Back away slowly while facing the animal (but don't make threatening eye contact) and continue to make yourself look large. If the cougar or wolf exhibits aggressive behavior, shout, throw rocks, and wave your arms violently. If a cougar attacks, try to stay standing and fight back as hard as you can. If a wolf attacks, curl into a ball and protect your face. Report sightings with the ranger station or by calling the Department of Fish and Wildlife (or 911 if it's an emergency).

## BEARS

Black bears live across the state, from the beach to the forest to subalpine territories of the mountains. Grizzly bears live in the North Cascades and in the Selkirk Mountains in northeastern Washington. Most campground bulletin boards will let you know if bears have been spotted in the area recently (or are likely to live there in general).

Do not approach bears of any species. If you see one, speak in a calm voice, and back away slowly while facing the bear (avoiding direct eye contact). Do not run, and do not yell. If the bear stays put, continue to back away slowly. If the bear charges you, plant your feet in a wide stance, and hold your ground (you cannot outrun a bear). Wave your arms overhead and speak in a soft, soothing, monotone voice. Do not scream or yell. If you have bear or pepper spray, be prepared to use it, but only if the bear gets to within 25 feet of you. Should a bear make contact, lie flat on your stomach or curl up on your side. Remain quiet and try not to panic, even if the bear attacks. Only when the bear has left the area should you get up to look for help.

Always check with the ranger station on what is required for food storage. For example, in some areas it's permissible to hang your food (12 feet high and 10 feet away from the nearest trunk). In other regions, you must have a bear canister (hanging food isn't allowed). Remember to store *all* scented items, including toiletries, food, trash, dishes that aren't fully washed, and lip balm. Some ranger stations have bear canisters available to borrow for free, but on busy weekends you can't count on them to be available. Consider investing in one. Report sightings with the ranger station or by calling the Department of Fish and Wildlife (or 911 if it's an emergency).

## DEER, ELK, AND MOOSE

Don't approach or feed any deer, elk, or moose you come across. Even if they seem calm, approaching may cause stress and agitate the animal, which could lead to aggressive behavior. If a moose were to charge, for example, they would likely kick their front legs forward to knock down the threat, then stomp with all four feet. Always keep a good distance—hooves and antlers are dangerous.

Washington is home to four main species of deer (white-tailed, black-tailed, Columbian white-tailed, and mule deer), two of elk (Roosevelt and Rocky Mountain), and one of moose

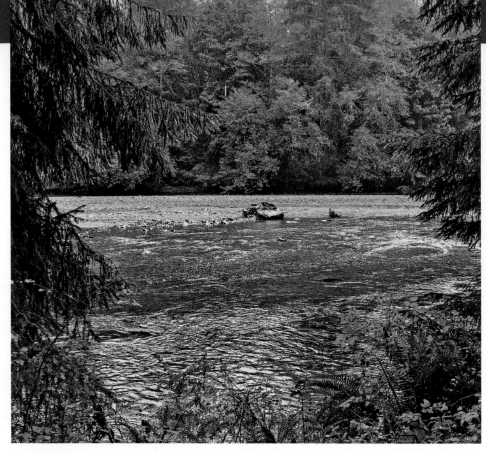

View of Queets River from Queets Campground (see page 37)

(Shiras). Depending on the species, deer can weigh up to 320 pounds. Elk can weigh up to 730 pounds, and moose top the scales at up to 1,000 pounds.

If any of these ruminants are grazing in the distance, you can usually enjoy watching from afar (without approaching). The biggest threat they pose (especially elk and deer) is to drivers at dusk and dawn, when the animals are most active and difficult to see on roadways.

## CAMPGROUND ETIQUETTE

Here are a few tips for creating good vibes with fellow campers and wildlife.

- **BE SURE TO CHECK IN,** pay your fee, and mark your site as directed. Don't make the mistake of grabbing a seemingly empty site that looks more appealing than your site. It could be reserved. If you're unhappy with the site you've selected, check with the campground host for other options.

- **BE SENSITIVE TO THE ENVIRONMENT** around you. Place tents on tent pad areas whenever provided. Be sure to place all garbage in a designated receptacle, or pack it out if none is available. Don't cut plants or move rocks to change the campsite.

- **YOU'RE A GUEST IN THE FOREST ANIMALS' HOME.** Give them space and respect but not your food. It's common for animals to wander through campsites, where they may be accustomed to the presence of humans (and our food). Try not to startle them with sudden movements or sounds. A surprised animal can be dangerous to you, to others, and to itself.

- **PLAN AHEAD.** Know your equipment, your ability, and the area where you are camping—and prepare accordingly. Weather, road, and wilderness conditions in Washington can change quickly. Call the regional forest ranger office to ask about road, trail, and weather advisories before you go. Carry necessary supplies for changes in weather or other conditions.

- **BE COURTEOUS TO OTHER CAMPERS,** hikers, bikers, and any other creatures you encounter.

- **FOLLOW THE CAMPGROUND AND REGIONAL RULES REGARDING FIRES.** Bring your own firewood instead of gathering it, and never burn trash.

## HAPPY CAMPING

There is nothing worse than a bad camping trip, especially because it is so easy to have a great time. To assist with making your outing a happy one, here are some pointers:

- **RESERVE YOUR SITE IN ADVANCE,** especially if it's a weekend or a holiday, or if the campground is wildly popular. Many prime campgrounds require at least a six-month lead time on reservations. If the reservation website allows bookings only 90 days in advance, be online exactly 90 days before your trip. Trust me. Some of the state's best campgrounds do not accept reservations, so have a backup campground (or two) in mind if you arrive and find all the sites full. Make a plan before you go. If you're already on the road, ranger stations can recommend nearby campgrounds.

- **COORDINATE GEAR** and expectations of difficulty (amenities or the lack thereof, physical exertion, and so on) with your camping buddies before you go. Make sure everyone knows what the weather and terrain will be like, what they need to bring, and expectations for getting in and out. If you're camping in a large group, don't duplicate equipment, but do plan to have backups of vital things like cookstoves, first aid kits, tarps, and lights. Carry what you need to have a good time, but don't turn the trip into a cross-country moving experience. Check that your gear is charged or fueled and working before you leave home.

- **DOWNLOAD A MAP OR OBTAIN A PAPER MAP** from the local ranger district office. The lure of the open road to the wilderness is less appealing when you're relying on Aunt Lucy's mental map from 20 years ago.

- **DRESS FOR THE SEASON.** Educate yourself on the temperature highs and lows of the specific part of the state you plan to visit, as temperatures can vary widely from your backyard to high-altitude mountains. Carry extra layers and an emergency kit in your car, including extra water (especially in eastern Washington), energy bars, extra flashlights, and emergency blankets.

- **PITCH YOUR TENT ON A LEVEL SURFACE,** and avoid low spots where water may pool at night. Use a tarp or specially designed footprint to thwart ground moisture and to protect the tent floor. Do a little site maintenance, such as picking up the small rocks and sticks that make sleep uncomfortable. Unless you're in a desert part of the state, plan for rain or excess condensation at night.

- **CONSIDER TAKING A SLEEPING PAD** if the ground makes you uncomfortable. Choose a pad that is full-length and thicker than you think you might need. This will not only keep your hips from aching on hard ground but will also help keep you warm. A wide range of thin, light, and inflatable pads is available at camping stores, and these are a much better choice than home air mattresses, which conduct heat away from the body and tend to deflate during the night.

- **PLAN TASTY MEALS** and bring everything you will need to prepare, cook, eat, and clean up. If you are not hiking to a primitive campsite, there is no real need to skimp on food due to weight. Bring an extra-large trash bag for your own refuse and to help keep the wilderness clean by packing out trash you find. Store food (including empty wrappers) and toiletries in your car at night to avoid attracting animal attention.

- **PLAN FOR TRIPS TO THE BATHROOM** if you tend to get up multiple times at night. Leaving a warm sleeping bag and stumbling around in the dark to find the restroom—whether it be a pit toilet, a fully plumbed comfort station, or just the woods—is not fun. Keep a flashlight and any other accoutrements you may need by the tent door, and know exactly where to head in the dark.

- **LOOK UP WHEN CHOOSING A CAMPSITE** or even just a spot to rest during a hike. Standing dead trees and storm-damaged living trees can pose a hazard to tent campers. These trees may have loose or broken limbs that could fall at any time.

## A WORD ABOUT BACKCOUNTRY CAMPING

Following these guidelines will increase your chances for a pleasant, safe, and low-impact interaction with nature.

- **PRACTICE "LEAVE NO TRACE" CAMPING ETHICS.** Adhere to the adages "Pack it in, pack it out" and "Take only pictures, leave only footprints." Visit lnt.org/learn/7-principles to learn more ways to enjoy the outdoors responsibly. Keeping Washington's wilderness healthy is a group effort. Plan to pack out some extra trash you may find on each trip. When others see you being generous and responsible, it will inspire them to do the same.

- **ALWAYS CHECK THE STATUS OF BURN BANS** before going, and bring a backpacking stove as a primary or backup. In Washington, open fires are permitted except during dry times, when the Forest Service may issue a fire ban. Many areas also prohibit collecting or cutting firewood.

- **HANG FOOD AWAY FROM BEARS** and other animals to prevent them from becoming introduced to (and dependent on) human food. Wildlife learns to associate backpacks and backpackers with easy food sources, thereby influencing their behavior.

- **BURY SOLID HUMAN WASTE** in a hole at least 6 inches deep and at least 200 feet away from trails and water sources; a trowel is basic backpacking equipment. Increasingly, however, the practice of burying human waste is being banned. You don't want to come across someone else's latrine next to your campsite, and they don't want to find yours. Using a portable latrine (which comes in various incarnations—basically a glorified plastic bag, given out by park rangers) may seem unthinkable at first, but it's really no big deal. Just bring an extra-large ziplock bag for additional insurance against structural failures.

## VENTURING AWAY FROM THE CAMPGROUND

If you go for a hike, bike ride, or other excursion into the wilderness, keep these precautions in mind:

- **ALWAYS CARRY FOOD AND WATER,** whether you are planning to go overnight or not. Food will give you energy, help keep you warm, and sustain you in an emergency until help arrives. Bring potable water, or treat water from a lake or stream by boiling or filtering it.

- **STAY ON DESIGNATED TRAILS.** Most hikers get lost when they leave the trail. Even on the most clearly marked trails, there is usually a point where you have to stop and consider which direction to head. If you become disoriented, don't panic. As soon as you think you may be off-track, stop, assess your current direction, and then retrace your steps back to the point where you went awry. If you have absolutely no idea how to continue, return to the trailhead the way you came in. Should you become completely lost and have no idea how to return to the trailhead, remaining in place along the trail and waiting for help is most often the best option for adults and always the best option for children.

- **BE ESPECIALLY CAREFUL WHEN CROSSING STREAMS.** Whether you are fording the stream or crossing on a log, make every step count. Look straight ahead, not down, for better balance. When fording a stream, avoid stepping on wet rocks, as they can be extremely slippery. Use a trekking pole or stout stick for balance, face upstream as you cross, and go slow. If a stream seems too deep to ford, turn back. Whatever is on the other side is not worth risking your life.

- **BE CAREFUL AT OVERLOOKS,** especially those by streams, which can undercut the overlook. Though these areas may provide spectacular views, they are hazardous. Washington has many hillsides that are prone to landslides after rains. Stay back from the edge of outcrops, and be absolutely sure of your footing: a misstep can mean a nasty and possibly fatal fall.

- **KNOW THE SYMPTOMS OF HYPOTHERMIA** and heat stroke. Shivering and forgetfulness are the two most common indicators of hypothermia. This can occur at any elevation, even in the summer. Wearing cotton clothing puts you especially at risk because cotton, when wet, wicks heat away from the body. To prevent hypothermia, dress in layers using synthetic clothing for insulation, use a cap and gloves to reduce heat loss, and protect yourself with waterproof, breathable outerwear. If symptoms arise, get the victim to shelter, a fire, hot liquids, and dry clothes or a dry sleeping bag. To avoid heatstroke, stay hydrated and take breaks. Signs of heatstroke include dizziness, headache, confusion, nausea, red skin, lack of sweating, and rapid heart rate. If symptoms arise, treat as a medical emergency, get to shade or seek help, rest, drink water, and apply wet cloths to the victim to help them cool down.

- **TAKE ALONG YOUR BRAIN.** A cool, calculating mind is the single most important piece of equipment you'll ever need on the trail. Think before you act. Watch your step. Plan ahead. Avoiding accidents before they happen is the best recipe for a rewarding and relaxing hike.

- **IF YOU PLAN ON HAVING AN ENHANCED EXPERIENCE IN NATURE** thanks to Washington's recreational marijuana laws, designate an experienced and/or sober person to be your safety monitor throughout your camping trip. Know the laws for where you can and cannot partake in smoking or edibles. For example, marijuana is never permitted on federal property, including national forests and national parks; possession on federal land can result in up to a year in prison. Don't hike or cook while intoxicated, as you may become lost easily or be more likely to have an accident. Remember that nature can be both awe inspiring and scary under the influence. Get to your destination, get set up for the night, then relax and enjoy.

## CHANGES

As with any guidebook, changes to the information provided in these pages are inevitable. It's a good idea to call ahead for the most updated report on the campground you've selected. We would appreciate knowing about any noteworthy changes you may come across.

# OLYMPIC PENINSULA AND SOUTHWESTERN WASHINGTON

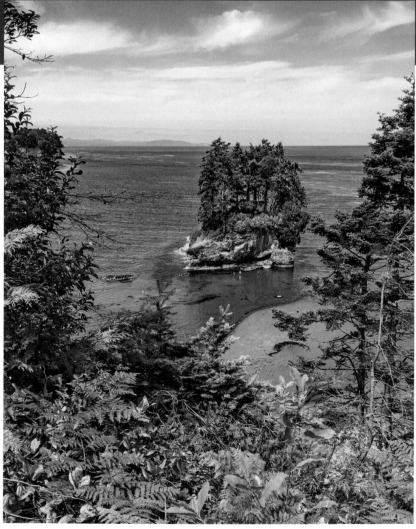

Salt Creek Recreation Area (see Lyre River Campground, page 31)

# 1

# Bruceport County Park Campground

Beauty ★★★★ Privacy ★★★★ Spaciousness ★★★★ Quiet ★★★★ Security ★★★★★ Cleanliness ★★★★★

*Here's an oasis in an otherwise tent-camping-parched region with views of Willapa Bay from your blufftop campsite.*

I had just about given up hope of finding a worthy campground on the Long Beach Peninsula. This is an area of Washington so unique in history, landscapes, economic activities, and environmental sensitivity that I felt it would be a loss not to have it represented from a tent-camping standpoint.

I had given myself several days to explore this far-southwestern region. I kept trying to give Cape Disappointment (formerly Fort Canby State Park) the benefit of the doubt, but it was too much of a three-ring circus for me. Other options were eliminated either for location, amenities, or not fitting the tent-camping profile—that is, for being too RV-oriented. Unfortunately, RVers are the recreation demographic to which much of this portion of the state caters.

Discouraged, I was retracing my route north from Long Beach on US 101, following the shoreline of Willapa Bay toward South Bend and Raymond, when I spied a sign for Bruceport County Park not far past the turnoff to Bay Center. Hmm, I thought. Never heard of this one before. I made a hard left into the entrance, and voilà!

The best sites look out over the wide, estuarine beauty of Willapa Bay.

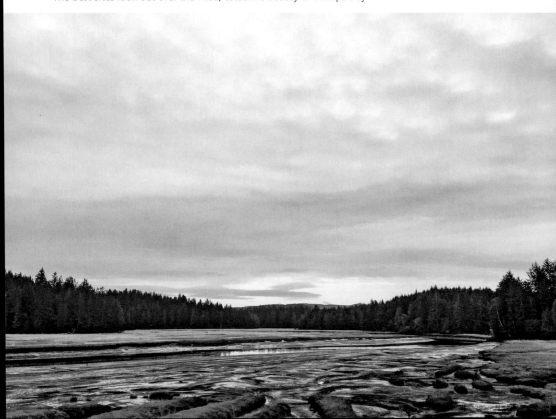

## KEY INFORMATION

**CONTACT:** 360-875-6611,
bruceportrvpark.com

**OPEN:** April–December

**SITES:** 23 standard, 8 with utilities, 8 primitive,
1 group area (up to 50 people)

**EACH SITE HAS:** Picnic table, fire pit with
grill; utility sites have water, electricity, and
sewage disposal

**ASSIGNMENT:** First come, first served, or by
reservation at 360-875-6611

**REGISTRATION:** On-site or by phone

**AMENITIES:** Restrooms with showers; day-
use area; covered group area with water,
electricity, barbecue pit, and wood-burning
stove; beach trail; camp host

**PARKING:** At individual sites

**FEE:** $20 standard, $25 utility (and site A6),
$15 hiker/biker (fees are for 4 people per
night, with a $2 fee for each additional
person), $50 group area (20–50 people)

**ELEVATION:** 500'

---

**RESTRICTIONS:**

**PETS:** On leash only

**FIRES:** In fire pits only

**ALCOHOL:** Permitted

**VEHICLES:** Trailers and RVs up to 30'

Allow me to introduce Bruceport County Park. Who knew? It's far from metropolitan centers, not listed specifically as a camping park on any maps or in any guidebooks, difficult to track down through online sources, and easily overlooked if you have your mind set on Long Beach as your destination. I regret that I may be bringing it kicking and screaming into the limelight, but a woman's gotta do what a woman's gotta do. And when you find a hidden gem—that's not really hidden at all, just a little removed and in the shadow of over-commercialized Long Beach—the find is as much fun as the camping experience itself.

The campground sits on 42 wooded acres of high-bank frontage along Willapa Bay and is a mix of individual tent sites; a stretch of hookup spaces (happily together away from most of the individual sites and guarding the 0.25-mile trail to the beach); several group areas (including a reservable covered one with a barbecue and woodstove); and a grassy primitive area for hikers (not sure how they would get here without a car), cyclists, and motorbikers. The drive in is far enough off US 101 that road noise is not a concern as far as I could hear—always something to consider when camping beside a main thoroughfare.

The best sites are rather obvious—those from A7 to G2 that line the bank and look out over the wide, estuarine beauty of Willapa Bay. Sites A7–A12 are more generously spaced. When you get back into the B section, they get tighter, but there is still plenty of vegetation between them, so it doesn't feel like they are intruding on each other. You'll be backed up to a gorgeous view anyway, and everyone else will be similarly distracted.

Bruceport is owned by the Pacific County Public Works Department and operated by camp hosts. If you are lucky, Jim and Janelle Long will still be holding down the joint when you arrive. Pacific County makes the rules and sets the fees, and the Longs keep everything operating smoothly (and have a couple of adorable dogs to help them out).

Bruceport isn't conveniently next door to Willapa Bay Wildlife Refuge or Leadbetter Point State Park. That said, it's not too far either—about an hour to an hour and 15 minutes by car. In fact, if you plan to venture to those places, making base camp at Bruceport allows you to more fully explore all the nooks and crannies of this unique part of Pacific County along the way.

A good place to start is the wildlife refuge headquarters, south on US 101 at mile marker 24 (a mile or so beyond the crossing of the Naselle River). It would be easy to spend your entire vacation educating yourself about the fragile, constantly shifting, wildlife-glutted wonders of this fascinating preserve. Definitely check out the newest addition at the headquarters: the Salmon Interpretive Trail, with art installations created by University of Washington art students.

If your interests lean more to local lore, head north to South Bend and visit the Pacific County Museum. Here you'll find out why the history of Bruceport reads like a historical docudrama. The historic Raymond Theater and the Northwest Carriage Museum are also nearby if you're on the lookout for more cultural destinations.

If you just want to play, good spots for beachcombing, kite flying, sea kayaking, and hiking surround you. The best sources I found for trip planning in the area are the Long Beach Peninsula Visitors Bureau (funbeach.com) and the Willapa Harbor Chamber of Commerce (willapaharbor.org).

## Bruceport County Park Campground

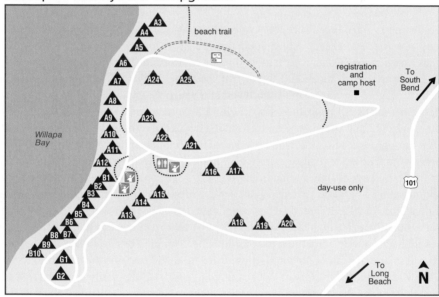

## GETTING THERE

From South Bend (approximately 30 miles south of Aberdeen), drive south 4 miles on US 101. The park entrance is on the right.

**GPS COORDINATES** N46° 41.017'  W123° 53.265'

# 2

# ⛺ Deer Park Campground

Beauty ★★★★★ Privacy ★★★★★ Spaciousness ★★★★★ Quiet ★★★★★ Security ★★★★★
Cleanliness ★★★★★

*This gem of a primitive, high-country bivouac sits inside Olympic National Park, with aerial-like views of the Olympic Range and alpine meadows.*

The sign reads NARROW WINDING ROAD NEXT 8 MILES. Thanks for the warning. Frankly, I don't even remember seeing that sign on the way up. But I sure had a few words for it on the way out—even took a picture to remind me.

Getting to Deer Park is kind of like applying for a government job: if you can get through the application, the job will be a breeze.

And that, Your Honor, is how I came to discover that I am a real chicken under certain backcountry road conditions.

Deer Park Road is definitely not for the faint of heart. Actually, the road condition is superb: fine, smooth, graded gravel; very few washboard ridges; no potholes. It's the altitude gain; the endless blind, hairpin, guardrail-challenged curves; the one-lane, I'm-over-as-far-as-I-can-go passage; and the sheer drop-offs that almost put me over the edge (pun fully intended). It was possibly the longest 8 miles of nerve-racking driving that I've done (you know, besides Hart's Pass). If you have any inclinations toward acrophobia or vertigo, let someone else drive. That's what I did on the way down. Thank you, Joan.

It's too bad I was so paralyzed on the way up because these 8 miles into the sky offer a new, stupendous view at every turn if you hit it on the kind of weekend we had. The entire

Deer Park Campground offers a panoramic vista of mountain peaks, green valleys, and blue sky.
photographed by *Ronald P. McDonald*

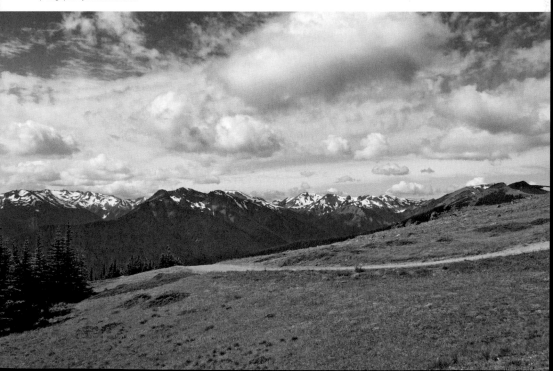

## KEY INFORMATION

**CONTACT:** 360-565-3130, nps.gov

**OPEN:** June–mid-October, depending on road conditions and snowmelt

**SITES:** 14

**EACH SITE HAS:** Picnic table, fire pit with grill

**ASSIGNMENT:** First come, first served

**REGISTRATION:** On-site

**AMENITIES:** Vault toilets, no water, ranger station nearby

**PARKING:** At individual sites

**FEE:** $15

**ELEVATION:** 5,400'

**RESTRICTIONS:**

**PETS:** On leash only

**FIRES:** In fire pits only, wood gathering prohibited

**ALCOHOL:** Permitted

**VEHICLES:** Trailers and RVs not permitted

Olympic Range lies before you as you momentarily burst out of the treeline. And you just know that if the scene is this good now, there's a possibility it might get better—which is exactly the case. Deer Park sits right at timberline just below the rounded summit of Blue Mountain and on the edge of glorious alpine meadows that simply shimmer in the hot August sun. A panoramic vista of razor-sharp mountain peaks, green valleys, and startling blue sky fills the eye. You find yourself taking deep breaths—partly from the rapid altitude gain to 5,400 feet—of the woody, earthy fragrance that wild places like this emit.

You'll also find yourself squinting a lot. This is a hat, sunglasses, and sunscreen zone. Bring plenty of water with you, too, as Deer Park has no potable water.

The campground itself is a bit of an oddball assortment of haphazardly situated campsites in three loops wrapped around the southwest slope. Loops A and B are more exposed to the elements, with jumbles of weathered timber adorning their front yards and not a lot of privacy between sites. Loop C offers the most forested setting, but it's also the throughway to the popular trailhead parking area and can be a bit busier than loops A and B.

We chose site 14 in Loop C mainly because there weren't too many options at 6 p.m. on a Thursday in August. It turned out to be a delightful spot—despite being the closest to the trailhead parking—mostly because it's a large space, its focus is internal (with the tent space at the lowest part of the site), and the trees provide considerable privacy.

The next morning we discovered the poorly marked site 13 straight across the parking lot from 14. We deduced that 13 is the best site in the camp, and that will be our choice on the next trip. It sits above the trailhead parking lot (which is also where its parking space is), and a narrow trail through the meadow leads up to it. Unlike at other sites, there is no campsite number marker. Site 13 is removed from the other campsites and affords the best blend of treeline protection and views of flowered meadows. An added plus is a morning cup of coffee at the picnic table drenched in luscious sunlight. You may encounter day hikers who think this is the trail to an outhouse, but you can direct them back to the toilet, where the three loops intersect.

Activities at Deer Park range from knocking around on the numerous trails, wildflower-identification sessions, and photo ops (when the quality of light presents itself) to nighttime stargazing and an informative chat with a park ranger (the ranger station is on the spur road just below where Deer Park Road crests).

Wildlife viewing is pretty easy too. Just sit in your campsite and watch the parade. We had a deer amble through several times while we were cooking dinner. A chipmunk boldly ransacked a bag of peanuts within seconds after we unpacked them. And those signs warning of bears? Take them seriously.

One last point: At this altitude, bring an extra layer of clothing even at the height of summer. Alpine nights are at least 10–15°F colder than nights at sea level. Even on a day that peaked somewhere above 90°F, we were reaching for the fleece by the time the sun set and kept our socks on in our sleeping bags.

## Deer Park Campground

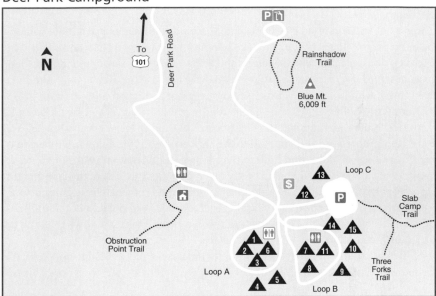

## GETTING THERE

From Port Angeles, drive 6 miles east on US 101 to Deer Park Road. Turn right and drive 18 miles to the campground. The last 9 miles are smooth gravel but very steep, with blind hairpin turns and no guardrails. Be extremely careful on the curves, drive slowly, and honk to announce your presence—better safe than sorry.

**GPS COORDINATES** N47° 56.882' W123° 15.591'

# 3

# Dungeness Recreation Area Campground

Beauty ★★★★★ Privacy ★★★★★ Spaciousness ★★★★ Quiet ★★★★ Security ★★★★ Cleanliness ★★★★

*This is the place from which to explore Dungeness Spit, one of the supreme natural wonders of Washington.*

Let me tell you about the day I almost didn't discover the rare beauty of Dungeness Recreation Area.

It was a hot and windy summer weekend. A friend and I had a last-minute wild notion to hop a ferry across Puget Sound and take our bicycles with us to Dungeness Spit. We had been told this was a special, unusual place, and we were eager to see firsthand if the description was deserved. We decided to explore by bicycle because the area is well suited to two-wheeled travel, with its flat, open expanses and pleasant country roads.

By midmorning the next day, we had battled our way by bicycle against a fierce head-wind from where we had camped the night before (we didn't know about Dungeness Recreation Area Campground at that point) to the park entrance. Windblown, we started down the narrow gravel road, following signs to the trailhead. Suddenly, an enormous automobile came careening up the road, filling up pretty much every usable inch of the lane and throwing up a shower of stones and a cloud of dust behind it. Fortunately, it ground to a halt before smashing us up against the roadside vegetation. A head poked out the driver's-side window and a voice growled, "No sense goin' down there. Don't know what all the fuss is about. I didn't see nothin' special 'bout that place."

Well, this fellow must have seen some pretty amazing sights in his life not to have been impressed with Dungeness Spit, but I can tell you we were very glad we ignored his advice.

View from the beach by the campground

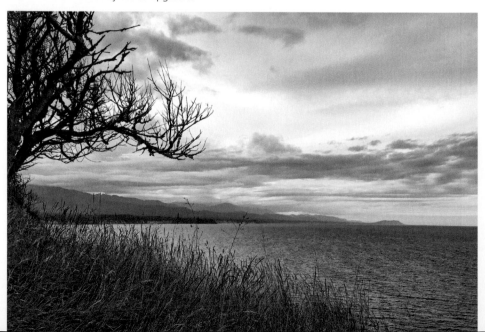

## KEY INFORMATION

**CONTACT:** 360-683-5847, ccpdu@olypen
.com, clallam.net/parks/dungeness.html

**OPEN:** May–September, daily, 6 a.m.–10 p.m.;
October–April, daily, 7 a.m.–9 p,m,

**SITES:** 66

**EACH SITE HAS:** Picnic table, fire pit,
shade trees

**ASSIGNMENT:** First come, first served;
reservations accepted for sites 34–66
February 1–October 31

**REGISTRATION:** At park information booth
(sunrise–sunset), online, or by phone

**AMENITIES:** Bathhouse with sinks, toilets,
showers, hot water; public telephone;
playground; firewood (for a small fee)

**PARKING:** At individual sites

**FEE:** $22 Clallam County resident, $25 non-
resident, $7 hiker/biker, $5 extra vehicle

**ELEVATION:** Sea level

**RESTRICTIONS:**

**PETS:** On leash only, no dogs on beach

**FIRES:** In fire pits only

**ALCOHOL:** Prohibited

**VEHICLES:** No size limit

We spent all afternoon exploring one of the supreme natural wonders of Washington, and I'm sure I spent at least a week recovering from a delightful, rare dose of too much sun and wind!

Dungeness Spit, the main attraction in Dungeness National Wildlife Refuge, is the longest natural sand spit in the country. Arcing nearly 7 miles into the Strait of Juan de Fuca on the Olympic Peninsula, this landform averages only 100 yards wide for its entire length.

Its outer (western) shore faces the open surf and uninterrupted winds, which cause driftwood to collect in jumbled masses like piles of giant bones. The inner shore—with smaller Graveyard Spit protruding from it—marks the boundary of Dungeness Bay. The innermost shoreline of this bay—actually an extremely shallow lagoon formed by Grave-yard Spit's finger—beckons thousands of migratory and wintering shorebirds that rest on the lush vegetation flourishing in these marshlike conditions. The oldest inland lighthouse in Washington sits 0.5 mile from the spit's end and warns off passing ships that can easily miscalculate their distance from barely submerged shoals.

The entire expanse of spits, tidelands, wetlands, landmarks, and adjoining surf forms Dungeness National Wildlife Refuge. While jurisdiction of the refuge belongs to the U.S. Department of Fish & Wildlife, Dungeness Recreation Area is in the hands of the Clallam County Parks Department. It's the largest of nine facilities managed by the county agency, most of which make use of the northern peninsula in some fashion.

The Dungeness Recreation Area campsites are well designed around two loops, affording ultimate privacy with dense undergrowth between sites. About a third of the sites are spaced along a high bluff that overlooks the Strait of Juan de Fuca and offer million-dollar views for the mere price of a campsite. On a clear night, look across to the twinkling lights of Victoria, British Columbia's capital, on the southern tip of Vancouver Island. Depending on the season and your timing, you may be able to enjoy this view complete with a dinner of world-famous Dungeness crab, caught in the local waters and cooked on your camp stove. Check with the Sequim Chamber of Commerce for information on where to find fresh local crab.

This area of the Olympic Peninsula lies within the rain shadow of the Olympic Mountains and, as a result, receives far less rain than just about any other area of western Washington. Rainfall averages about 18 inches per year (compared with Seattle's 35–50).

Thanks to the moderate year-round climate, the campground is open all year—but accepts reservations only from February 1 to October 31, and only for some of its sites. Summer can be quite busy, so you may want to try the off-season.

In addition to the ever-popular beachcombing, park activities include horseback riding (using a separate equestrian trail and unloading area), game-bird hunting in designated areas, and good old-fashioned picnicking along the bluff, with its stunning view.

## Dungeness Recreation Area Campground

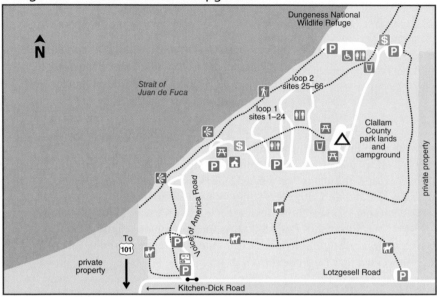

## GETTING THERE

From Sequim, drive 5 miles west on US 101 to Kitchen-Dick Road. Turn right (north) and drive 3 miles, watching for signs to the recreation area campground and entrance. The entrance is on the left just past the 90-degree turn where Kitchen-Dick becomes Lotzgesell Road.

**GPS COORDINATES** N48° 07.831' W123° 11.778'

# 4

# Fairholme Campground

Beauty ★★★★★ Privacy ★★★ Spaciousness ★★★★ Quiet ★★★ Security ★★★ Cleanliness ★★★★★

*Enjoy views of brilliant blue water from the comfort of your campsite.*

If you're all about beauty tucked away in a Douglas-fir forest beside an exquisite lake, you're going to be all about Fairholme Campground. The campground sits on the shores of Lake Crescent, which often appears a brilliant deep blue and sometimes a teal green. If you haven't yet experienced this lake, there isn't a better way to do so than by setting up your temporary home at its edge.

The campground is bigger than some in this book—with a whopping 87 sites to choose from—but what it lacks in privacy, it makes up for in sheer natural wonder. Arranged in three loops, the sites are spaced generously. Each includes a fire pit and picnic table. Sites range from somewhat open (staggered among old-growth trees along the sloping hill down to the lake) to slightly more private (higher up on the hillside, not as close to the lake, but with a little more vegetation between sites). Even with a clear view of your fellow campers, you will likely be magnetized by the view of the lake if you're lucky enough to see it from your picnic table. I recommend opting for a walk-in site (53–59) for premium proximity to the lake. Most of these sites have animal-proof storage lockers for your convenience—a pretty nice perk for having to walk your gear in a little ways (50–100 yards).

Walk-in sites on the shore of Lake Crescent

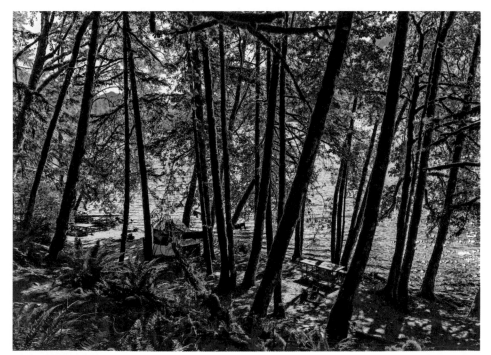

**CONTACT:** 360-374-6131, nps.gov

**OPEN:** May–September (but check each year, as the dates tend to shift around a little)

**SITES:** 87

**EACH SITE HAS:** Picnic table, fire pit with grill

**ASSIGNMENT:** First come, first served

**REGISTRATION:** Self-registration on-site

**AMENITIES:** Flush toilets, potable water, animal-proof storage lockers, dump station ($10 per use of dump station)

**PARKING:** At individual sites

**FEE:** $20

**ELEVATION:** 700'

**RESTRICTIONS:**

**PETS:** On leash only

**FIRES:** In fire pits only

**ALCOHOL:** Permitted

**VEHICLES:** RVs up to 21'

No matter which site you're in, you'll want to leave it to go for a walk along the lake or to enjoy a dip at Fairholme Beach. The views of the lake and the mountains are incredible! If you plan to jump in and enjoy the benefits of the freezing—and I do mean very, very cold—waters, bring a towel. Even a small chamois or microfiber number will really help you out. You cannot rely on the heat or sunshine of July or August to warm you up, as many of the trails are shaded, and the slightest of breezes will chill you to the core—just trust me on this one. The water temperature comes in at about 44°F no matter the time of year. It usually takes a couple of minutes to get used to it, but then you'll get the chance to practice your butterfly stroke in one of the most beautiful places you'll ever swim. Hands down, it's worth it.

A small boat launch is here as well if you prefer to enjoy the water without being completely submerged (the Fairholme store a mile away has boat rentals during summer). And if you prefer more walking and less swimming, I recommend a 10-minute drive down the road to Marymere Falls for a 0.5-mile hike with waterfalls, or go for the 10-mile hike at Barnes Creek. You could also do Aurora Creek, or simply hang out, picnic, and explore Lake Crescent Lodge.

One could argue that the beauty of Lake Crescent Lodge is the reason we have Olympic National Park to begin with. While the Olympic Forest had already been established and protected thanks to President Grover Cleveland in 1897, it wasn't until 1937 that Lake Crescent Lodge hosted its most distinguished guest, President Franklin D. Roosevelt. The year following his tour of the beautiful Olympic range, Roosevelt signed Olympic National Park into existence. I like to think his stay at Lake Crescent is what gave him the extra nudge. Cabins built in subsequent years were named the Roosevelt cabins.

But who needs cabins when you have a tent?

If you're sitting around your campsite and wondering how the water looks so emphatically blue and so crystal clear, it's because of the lack of nitrogen. Without algae growth, the depths of Lake Crescent are yours to gaze into—depths of around 600 feet! Of course you won't be able to see quite that far down, but in some places it's said to have clarity of up to 60 feet, which is still very impressive. The lake is glacier carved, like many lakes in the Northwest, and the depth has been disputed for years. Unfortunately, depth-measuring technology has been unable to confirm the rumors of 1,000 feet.

Like nearby Lyre River, the isolation of the lake has spawned unique species. The Beardslee and Crescenti trout are not found anywhere else in the world. Their declining population has incited a movement to protect them, and more regulations have been put in place to prevent removing them from the area. That said, it's still legal to fish at Lake Crescent, and some people claim that fly-fishing is the way to go here.

If you get a clear night, you're bound to see plenty of stars. If your stay is especially auspicious, you may even see the Milky Way reflected in the still water of the lake.

## Fairholme Campground

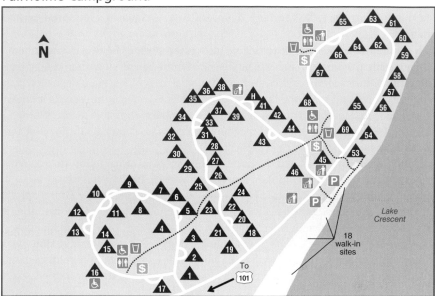

## GETTING THERE

From Port Angeles, take US 101 west about 25 miles. Turn right into the campground, just before Camp David Jr. Road.

**GPS COORDINATES** N48° 04.126'  W123° 55.229'

# 5

# ⛺ Hoh Rain Forest Campground

Beauty ★★★★★ Privacy ★★★★ Spaciousness ★★★★ Quiet ★★★★ Security ★★★ Cleanliness ★★★★★

*One of only three temperate rainforests in the world, this is a unique and therefore popular destination, especially with hikers. You may want to visit in the off-season.*

The first thing you'll notice as you drive up Hoh River Road toward the Hoh Rain Forest Visitor Center and Campground is just how green everything is around you. Even the small bits of sun that manage to leak through the nearly impenetrable canopy of foliage seem to have a green tinge.

The second thing you'll notice is the pale gray-green shrouds of mosses and lichens that drape ghoulishly from tree branches. The weight of these hangers-on often causes limbs to snap under the stress.

Third, as you stand amid the hushed majesty of this primeval forest, you'll notice the most insidious and perpetual characteristic of a temperate rainforest: the steady *plink! plink! plink!* as droplet after droplet of moisture makes its small but significant contribution to this fascinating, self-sustaining ecosystem.

The Hoh Rain Forest has had the good fortune to have remained in its original state for thousands of years, thanks to the vision of a few men around the turn of the century who recommended the preservation of the Roosevelt elk habitat. Their efforts led first to the creation of the Olympic Forest Reserve, then to Mount Olympus National Monument (under Teddy Roosevelt), and finally to Olympic National Park (under Franklin Roosevelt).

You'll notice as you make your way around Olympic Peninsula to the Hoh entrance that logging has been rampant up to the park boundary. Examples of the colossal trees that once blanketed the western slopes of the Olympic Mountains all the way to the coast have,

A tent is nearly camouflaged in a private site among the Hoh Rain Forest's ferns.

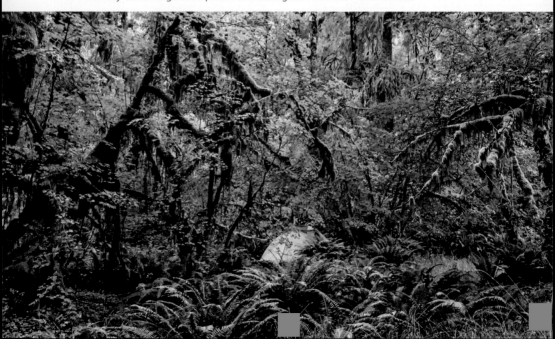

## KEY INFORMATION

**CONTACT:** 360-374-6925, Olympic National Park visitor center; 360-452-4501, park headquarters; 360-565-3131, road and weather conditions (updated twice daily); nps.gov

**OPEN:** Year-round

**SITES:** 78

**EACH SITE HAS:** Picnic table, fire pit with grill

**ASSIGNMENT:** First come, first served; no reservations

**REGISTRATION:** Self-registration at bulletin board next to restrooms

**AMENITIES:** Restrooms with flush toilets, sinks; potable water; animal-proof storage lockers; summer naturalist program; visitor center

**PARKING:** At individual sites

**FEE:** $20

**ELEVATION:** 578'

---

**RESTRICTIONS:**

**PETS:** On leash only, not permitted on trails or in public buildings

**FIRES:** In fire pits only

**ALCOHOL:** Permitted

**VEHICLES:** Trailers and RVs up to 21', no hookups

**OTHER:** Feeding birds or animals prohibited, permits required for overnight hikes

---

fortunately, been preserved within the park's borders. Four of the nine world-record holders are along the Hoh River and its forks. Check at the visitor center for their exact locations.

The Hoh Rain Forest Visitor Center and Campground will probably be one of the busiest facilities you'll come across in this book. The rainforest attracts visitors from all over the world, but its uniqueness warrants inclusion in this guide. Summer sees the most visitors, naturally, but the park is open year-round, so you may want to plan a visit in the off-season.

Temperatures are never really hot or cold at any time of the year in the Hoh Valley, but spending time here in seasons other than summer and late spring means limiting your hiking to low elevations. The Hoh River Valley itself is a grand off-season walk, with round-trip distances up to 18 miles without significant altitude gain. In the immediate vicinity of the visitor center are three short nature trails of varying lengths that feature fine examples of rainforest vegetation. One often sees elk on these short trips.

For more energetic backpackers coming to the Hoh in summer, Hoh River Trail is the most popular access to Mount Olympus. If you are planning to camp overnight on your way to Blue Glacier (39 miles round-trip from the Hoh Rain Forest Visitor Center), you're required to obtain a Wilderness Camping Permit, which you can get in person at the Wilderness Information Center in Port Angeles or at the Hoh Visitor Center.

It's 18.5 miles to Blue Glacier at the base of the east peak of Mount Olympus. The Hoh trail also connects with other major (trunk) trails in the park. Backcountry permits are required for any overnight travel on the trails. Check with a park ranger for further information if you plan extended backpacking trips within the park. The nearest spot for supplies is Westward Hoh (a resort 5.6 miles from the intersection with US 101).

You are advised not to attempt boating or swimming in the Hoh River because it moves rapidly and is very cold and often jammed with logs. Fishing is, however, one safe option, and a list of regulations is available at the visitor center.

The campground is set between two bends in the river, giving campers the most river frontage possible. The best sites will be those in loops A and C, which are closest to the river.

Unless the river is at flood stage, just sitting and watching the flow of water can be a mesmerizing and soothing activity. If the river floods, there's a good chance you won't get this far up the road. Ongoing efforts attempt to keep the slides and washouts to a minimum. In 2004, the rambunctious Hoh was retrofitted using logjams to keep it from ruining the road system along it. In 2016, Upper Hoh Road closed for a chunk of the year after storm damage.

It's worth noting that the drive to the Hoh River Valley is easily several hours by car from metropolitan Puget Sound. Unless you already plan to be on the peninsula, this is a long weekend outing.

## Hoh Rain Forest Campground

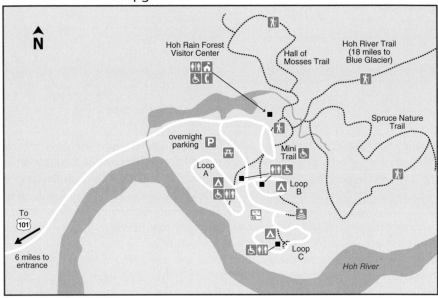

## GETTING THERE

Whether you are coming from the north or the south, take US 101 around the Olympic Peninsula to the west side of Olympic National Park. Turn east onto Upper Hoh Road, about 18 miles south of the town of Forks; the campground is at the end of the road. The driving distance from Seattle by way of Olympia is roughly 200 miles. By way of Washington ferries to Winslow or Kingston, the road distance is about 145 miles. Ferry crossings take about half an hour.

**GPS COORDINATES** N47° 51.589'  W123° 56.052'

# 6

# Lyre River Campground

Beauty ★★★ Privacy ★★★★ Spaciousness ★★★★ Quiet ★★★★ Security ★★★ Cleanliness ★★★★★

*Free camping on the Olympic Peninsula is almost unheard of, but here's one that's also off the beaten path and only a short distance from salt water.*

Obscured by the clamor for the Sol Duc River, Lake Crescent, Neah Bay, Lake Ozette, the Black Ball Ferry to Victoria, Salt Creek Recreation Area—you name it—the Lyre River Campground is one of the Department of Natural Resources (DNR) hidden gems that has everything going for it and nobody promoting it, until now.

For starters, and thanks to the generous contribution of the DNR (although this could change very soon), it's free. Second, it's an agate's throw from the pebble-strewn beaches of the Strait of Juan de Fuca. Third, it's just far enough outside the Olympic National Park radar to get conveniently overlooked. Plus, it's easily confused with Lyre River Park (a privately run resort that must have spent every extra dollar it made to get written up in just about every guidebook and on every website that lists recreational accommodations on the north Olympic Peninsula). Finally, the Lyre River at its origins with Lake Crescent happens to be home to a species of trout found nowhere else on earth! How's that for a heavy-hitting package?

On to more serious matters. Like camping.

Nestled in private pockets of Olympic coastal vegetation, the 11 campsites at Lyre River are close enough to the river for one to hear and hum along with its melody. The DNR has

Campsites at Lyre River are nestled in pockets of coastal vegetation.

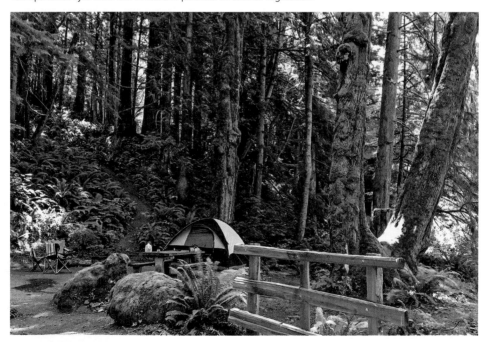

## KEY INFORMATION

**CONTACT:** 360-374-6131, dnr.wa.gov
/olympicpeninsula

**OPEN:** Year-round

**SITES:** 11

**EACH SITE HAS:** Picnic table, fire pit with grill

**ASSIGNMENT:** First come, first served

**REGISTRATION:** Not necessary

**AMENITIES:** Vault toilets (1 ADA accessible),
picnic shelter with fireplace, potable water

**PARKING:** At individual sites

**FEE:** Free to camp; Discover Pass required
to park ($11.50 per day or $35 for an
annual pass)

**ELEVATION:** Sea level

---

**RESTRICTIONS:**

**PETS:** On leash only

**FIRES:** In fire pits only

**ALCOHOL:** Permitted

**VEHICLES:** Trailers and RVs not
recommended

---

not outdone itself with elaborate upgrades, and all is maintained in a very natural state (read: primitive). There's a picnic shelter identical to every one I've seen at other DNR sites, and potable water—an amenity you tend not to expect in rustic surroundings—is available from a spigot at the north end of the campground.

There's no doubt that Lyre's main allure is its coastal location providing saltwater access. Rock collecting and tidepool marveling could keep you busy all day. But eventually the tide rushes in, and unless you like getting very wet, you have to find alternative entertainment.

This calls for some upland meandering. Destinations are every direction, but some of the more notable ascents (and easily managed in a few hours) are Striped Peak Lookout, over at Salt Creek Recreation Area; Spruce Railroad Trail, hugging Lake Crescent's north shore; and the more challenging Mount Storm King, which rises high above Lake Crescent on the Olympic National Park boundary. You might also venture to Murdock Beach at low tide to search for agates or make your way to Tongue Point if tidepools are what you're after.

Lyre River, not far from the confluence with Susie Creek

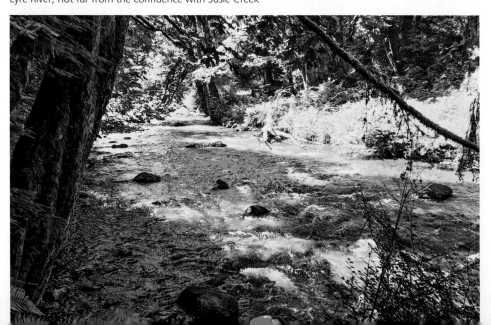

As noted earlier, the headwaters of the Lyre at Lake Crescent are, for reasons unknown, the singular spawning ground for prized Beardslee rainbow trout, or bluebacks, as the locals call them. The fate of this rare species, native only to Lake Crescent, has in the past several years come under the scrutiny of Washington Trout (essentially a well-intentioned nonprofit fish-police organization). At its urging, the national park has agreed to a catch-and-release-only program as the first critical step in saving the fish. This puts Lyre River on the map, so to speak, for anglers who pay attention to these kinds of developments. To most fishing enthusiasts, however, and fortunately for the Beardslee rainbow, Lyre River is popular for its salmon and steelhead runs. The campground obliges with an area that accommodates the activity accordingly. A fishing platform!

For all its primitiveness, Lyre River embraces a barrier-free principle, with one campsite, all facilities, the parking lot, and the path leading to the campsite all wheelchair accessible. Between this accommodation of the challenged recreationist and the efforts being made to restore the endangered trout population, we can be proud that public agencies are taking this kind of initiative, even in such low-impact areas as Lyre River.

It's enough to make me want to strum a tune. Now, where did I put my lyre?

## Lyre River Campground

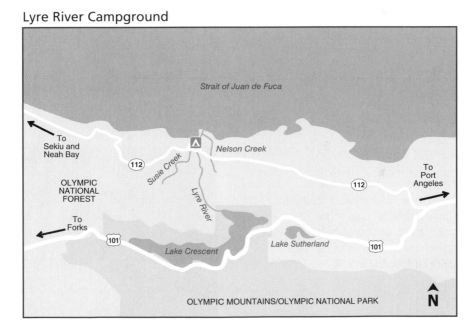

## GETTING THERE

From Port Angeles, go west on US 101 roughly 5 miles to the turn for WA 112 (Sekiu/Neah Bay). Head west on WA 112, and look for Lyre River Road (paved) between mileposts 46 and 47. Turn right, drive 0.5 mile, and turn left into the campground. Don't confuse this campground with the privately owned and operated Lyre River Resort and RV Park. The resort is farther west on West Lyre River Road and has signage that can be misleading.

**GPS COORDINATES** N48° 09.142′ W123° 49.842′

# 7

# Mora Campground

Beauty ★★★★ Privacy ★★★★ Spaciousness ★★★★ Quiet ★★★★★ Security ★★★ Cleanliness ★★★★

*No other public campground in Washington brings you so close by car to wilderness beaches that are accessible only by foot.*

Grab your Gore-Tex for this one! We're heading for the wet and wild (or should I say wetter and wilder?) side of Olympic National Park to some of the last stretches of coastal wilderness left in the contiguous United States.

Mora Campground, part of a network of well-attended Olympic National Park facilities, is among the elite when it comes to its location: only a mile or so from the Pacific Ocean. For 57 unspoiled and challenging miles—from the Quillayute River north to the boundary of the Makah Indian Reservation, and south to the legendary Hoh River—the ocean frontage features numerous protruding headlands, swirling tidepools, crashing surf, and stalwart "sea stacks."

For many years, this outpost of civilization was an active trading port for ships from Seattle. When neither roads nor rail materialized, boat-only access kept Mora safe from further development.

In 1990 a major oil spill near Cape Flattery (the northwesternmost piece of land in the lower 48 states) cast a pall over certain sections of the coastal parklands. It will never be the same, but it seems that much of the oil was controlled and scooped up, thanks to the quick response of various agencies.

Fortunately, this is still one of the truly remarkable and entrancing spots in the country, perhaps even in the world. The blend of natural geography, cultural influence, and historical record are a powerful combination. The weather-beaten Washington coast can be formidable even when there are no storms. This is a place where rain slickers, wool sweaters, waterproof footwear, and a hat you can hold on to are very much in order at any time of the year. Western winds hit the coast unchecked and work the surf into a foaming frenzy. As a result, the shape of the coastline is forever changing.

Mora Campground is a relatively large complex compared to other Olympic Park accommodations. Situated at sea level, it is open all year and is an ideal choice for off-season travel. Actually, weather-wise, winter and early spring can be some of the best times to be on the Washington coast. You

Site 34 at Mora Campground

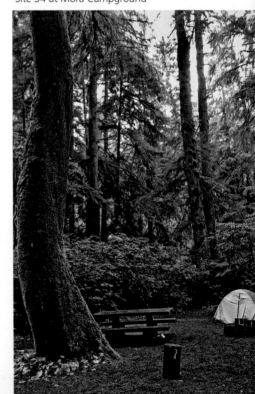

## KEY INFORMATION

**CONTACT:** 360-374-5460, olym_visitor
_center@nps.gov

**OPEN:** Year-round

**SITES:** 94 (1 walk-in)

**EACH SITE HAS:** Picnic table, fire pit with grill

**ASSIGNMENT:** First come, first served;
no reservations

**REGISTRATION:** Self-registration on-site

**AMENITIES:** Bathhouse with toilets, sinks,
running water; drinking water; animal-
proof storage lockers

**PARKING:** At individual sites

**FEE:** $20

**ELEVATION:** Sea level

**RESTRICTIONS:**

**PETS:** On leash only

**FIRES:** In fire pits only

**ALCOHOL:** Permitted

**VEHICLES:** Trailers and RVs up to 21', no
vehicles allowed off park roads

**OTHER:** Permits required for extended hikes
into backcountry

will have an opportunity to watch migrating gray whales on their way to Southern California and Mexico.

The campground consists of five loops. Sites are so spacious among the giant firs and cedars, and shrouded from each other by the dense, low-growing foliage, that even at its busiest, Mora offers campers side-by-side solitude. Only the most monstrous RVs poke out from their parking spaces in what seems like embarrassed apology.

If time allows, be sure to take a full tour of all the loops before deciding on your site. You may want to park and enjoy the tour on foot. This will give you the best sense of the place and a good firsthand analysis of where you're going to make your home for the next few days. Plus, the grandeur of the land loses something with motor vehicles puttering around. It's too bad there isn't some system to shuttle campers in and out of Mora by boat, long canoe, or horseback. These seem much more fitting modes of travel here.

Since Mora is first come, first served (like most of the developed campgrounds in Olympic National Park), the best sites fill up fast—but in this campground, the definition of "best" may depend on the camper. My first choice would be any of the sites in loop E on the river side. But perhaps the best site in the entire campground is what used to be the group camp. Severe flooding has restructured the site to be walk-in only; it can accommodate up to six people (two tents maximum). It sits alone at the end of loop D on a low bluff above the Quillayute River surrounded by trees and shrubbery. The walk is down a wide, well-maintained path, which was softened with fresh cedar chips when I was there.

Ocean access from Mora is 2 miles beyond the campground at Rialto Beach, where there is ample parking for a day hike or an extended trek. Permits are required if you plan to stay on the wilderness beach overnight (see Rialto Beach Campground, page 40). A word of warning: Coastal hiking requires a tide table at all times of the year. Many of the points, bluffs, heads, and capes are covered at high tide, and you'll need to either wait out the tide or, where possible, go overland to continue. Even the inland routes can be muddy and treacherous, so make sure you have good traction on your shoes or boots. The "Strip of Wilderness" brochure available at the Mora Ranger Station is full of information about the pleasures and pitfalls of coastal hiking.

For other options in this part of Olympic National Park and the surrounding national forest, check at either the Mora station or information stations along US 101—there's one north of Forks and one at Kalaloch.

One last word: The Indian reservations that border the park along the coast are private lands. Be respectful of this fact.

## Mora Campground

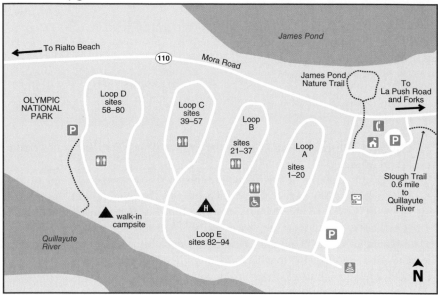

## GETTING THERE

Whether you are coming from the north or the south, take US 101 around the Olympic Peninsula to the town of Forks (125–200 miles from Seattle, depending on which route you take). About 1 mile north of Forks, turn west onto La Push Road (WA 110) and drive about 10 miles to Mora Road. Turn right onto Mora Road and follow the signs to the campground.

**GPS COORDINATES** N47° 55.077'  W124° 36.449'

# 8

# Queets Campground

Beauty ★★★★ Privacy ★★★★ Spaciousness ★★★★★ Quiet ★★★★ Security ★★★★ Cleanliness ★★★★★

*One of the Olympic Peninsula's lush green oases, this primitive campground has it all when it comes to trees and rivers.*

Whether I'm on the coast or in the rainforest, I cannot seem to get enough of camping on the Olympic Peninsula. I thought I already knew my go-to spots in this neck of the woods, but a friend turned me on to Queets Campground. She assured me this was a premium stopover on the way to the coast, and I'm pleased to report she was absolutely right—Queets is a gem.

Here's the thing: It's surrounded by stands of giant spruce and hemlock and nestled along the Queets River. It feels quaint and homey. The campsites are large, and everything feels secluded.

Because it's in the rainforest, it can be damp, so bring all the appropriate layers and gear to make your visit a comfortable one should the clouds decide to impart a couple of inches of rain. Plus, even when it's raining, hiking is still the premium activity in a rainforest. Rather than a mountaintop view, the dense forest will be your focus. Let's take the Queets Campground Loop for starters. The trail is just 2.8 miles and mostly flat the whole way. There are ferns, oxalis, hemlock, and giant spruce trees. You'll see nurse logs and new

A spacious rainforest campsite

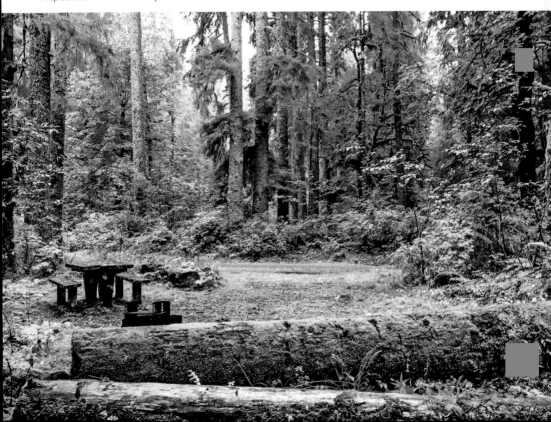

## KEY INFORMATION

**CONTACT:** 360-374-6131, nps.gov

**OPEN:** Year-round

**SITES:** 20

**EACH SITE HAS:** Picnic table, fire pit with grill

**ASSIGNMENT:** First come, first served

**REGISTRATION:** Not necessary

**AMENITIES:** Vault toilets, no water, no hookups

**PARKING:** At individual sites

**FEE:** $15

**ELEVATION:** 183'

---

**RESTRICTIONS:**

**PETS:** On leash only, not permitted on trails

**FIRES:** In fire pits only

**ALCOHOL:** Permitted

**VEHICLES:** Small trailers only (limited side clearance)

**OTHER:** Permits and bear canisters required for extended hikes into backcountry

growth, and the river is at the center of it all. You may hear or see owls, frogs, squirrels, and birds aplenty. Dogs are not allowed on the trails, though they're welcome at the campground if someone holds down the fort there.

Sam's River Loop is another worthy little hike (about 3 miles). Because this area is less trafficked than other spots in the park, you should have a pleasant time hiking any nearby trail. There shouldn't be crowds, and the forest will be beautiful rain or shine. (Even if it's sunny, you'll likely be walking in the shade.) You'll pass big-leaf maples, hemlock, and spruce here too—and all the moss you could ever hope for. The moss here on the peninsula always makes me feel like I'm walking in a fairy tale.

If you need a longer walk, Queets River Trail is 16.2 miles and has a lot of elevation gain. This hike includes fording Sam's River and Queets River, which can be dangerous depending on the water levels. Don't attempt to cross these rivers until late summer or early fall, and always use your best judgment. If there has been a big storm lately, it might be wise to turn back.

At the campground, the river is wide and flat. It feels peaceful, and the vegetation is lush and green on the banks. If boating is more your thing than hiking, come to Queets when the water level is high. Paddle the Queets River from the campground and enjoy Class II and III rapids to Sam's Rapid and down to the Hartzell boat launch, where you'll want to get out. I haven't kayaked it myself, but if you're experienced, it shouldn't be much of a challenge, and if you're a novice, be sure to keep your eyes open for logjams, as they can create some serious hazards on this route no matter the time of year. Being in the river is a great way to experience the rainforest.

If you head to the wilderness primarily to find solitude, Queets is the perfect place for you. It has only 20 campsites, and this area of the rainforest is less visited than others. Queets is not too far from more popular destinations, like Kalaloch, Quinault, and Hoh, but this outer edge of Olympic National Park doesn't seem to be on anyone's radar (which is perhaps why I didn't get myself here sooner). The remoteness is almost tangible.

The campsites are big and feel very open. At some sites you may feel a little snug next to your neighbor, but vegetation as well as low-hanging moss-covered branches create a bit of privacy. Most sites are situated at the river's edge, which makes for a great soundscape as you sleep. I like sites 2 and 4, but any of them provide a little paradise. Watch for puddles as you drive the loop if it's been extra wet lately. The ground is always at risk of being damp, and you don't want to end up in the wettest spot.

I should mention that the ranger station is not likely to be open, even in "peak season." With the small number of people venturing to this corner of the park, it's probably not worth it to staff the place. The road here is windy, partly because it had to be rerouted after a landslide in 2005, which could be part of the reason people keep to the bigger campgrounds. I would venture to guess there are more elk at Queets Campground than people. Keep your eyes out for them—they might be off in the woods, nibbling the fruit from an old homesteader's abandoned orchard.

## Queets Campground

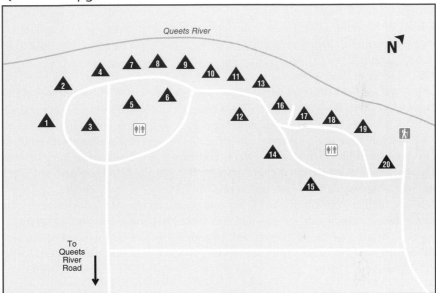

## GETTING THERE

From Amanda Park, drive west on US 101 North about 10.5 miles. Turn right at the Upper Queets entrance to Olympic National Park (onto West Boundary Road). Continue about 6 miles, then bear left; the road will become NF 2405. After about 4 miles, bear left again, onto NF 2433. Then left onto NF 2410. After another mile or so, turn right onto Queets River Road. Queets Campground is well marked with signage.

**GPS COORDINATES** N47° 36.862' W124° 02.121'

# 9

# Rialto Beach Campground

Beauty ★★★★★ Privacy ★★★★★ Spaciousness ★★★★★ Quiet ★★★★★ Security ★★ Cleanliness ★★★★★

**This is oceanside camping at its finest—and the best possible introduction for those new to backpacking.**

The majesty of the open ocean, the impressive windblown trees, and the gigantic drift logs make this spot feel larger than life. Rialto Beach is one of my favorite places in Washington. I love anywhere along the coast, but Rialto has the perfect balance of easy-to-get-to while still feeling extremely remote. It's a long haul from Seattle, at about four hours without traffic (no matter which route you take), but it's worth it for even a short weekend (though a long weekend is preferred). If you've only been car camping, or maybe to a walk-in site at another campground, Rialto Beach is a perfect introduction to backpacking. I like to call it "baby backpacking."

Many people exploring the coast use this as a day-use area (and you can too if you're staying up the road at Mora Campground), so don't be thrown off by the number of cars in the parking lot. Also, don't leave any valuables in your car. You'll need a permit and a bear canister for this light trek, both available at the Port Angeles Wilderness Information Center (WIC) if you drive the northern route. When I was here last summer, self-registration permits were available on-site, which you need to mail in after your camping adventure. That said, it's your responsibility to have a permit for overnight backcountry camping. You can call the WIC ahead of time with questions.

So you've parked your car, you've loaded your pack, and you've filled your bear canister; it's time to hike to your campsite. I should emphasize that you're required to keep all food as well as all fragrant items—like deodorant, toothpaste, and any empty food packaging—in a bear canister. I recommend buying one before you leave your home base, but it's possible

From the parking lot at Rialto Beach, crest the hill for a better view of Little James Island to the south. Hike north to find your campsite beyond Ellen Creek.

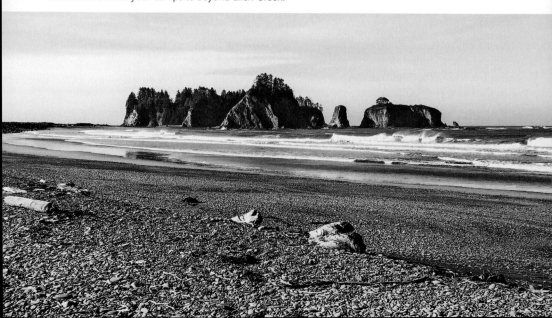

## KEY INFORMATION

**CONTACT:** 360-565-3100, nps.gov

**OPEN:** Year-round

**SITES:** Beach camping between Ellen Creek and Hole-in-the-Wall; groups limited to 12 people

**EACH SITE HAS:** Primitive, some with established tent space or fire pit

**ASSIGNMENT:** First come, first served

**REGISTRATION:** On-site or via mail (addressed envelopes are provided at the campground); Wilderness Camping Permit available at the Wilderness Information Center in Port Angeles

**AMENITIES:** Vault toilets by parking lot, bury waste 6–8" deep and 200' from campsites and water sources

**PARKING:** At trailhead

**FEE:** $8 per person, free for age 15 and under

**ELEVATION:** Sea level

---

**RESTRICTIONS:**

**PETS:** On leash only during day, camping with pets prohibited

**FIRES:** In fire rings or on the beach (away from tree roots), only driftwood gathering permitted

**FOOD:** All food, garbage, and fragrant items must be stored in park-approved bear canisters (or in your car)

**ALCOHOL:** Permitted

**VEHICLES:** Small trailers only (limited side clearance)

**OTHER:** Backcountry wilderness permits required for overnight stays

to find one at an outdoor store along the drive, or nab one of the limited supply at the WIC. Don't forget to pack a rope with which to hang it from a tree branch. If you don't have a bear canister, you must leave your food in your car. Don't worry—it's mostly raccoons you're protecting yourself from. And don't worry if you didn't get ahold of a bear canister—it's still possible to camp overnight. You'll just have to hike in and out to eat your meals. Bonus: You'd get to use the restroom as well.

The hike from the parking lot to the area where you're allowed to camp is only 0.8 mile. If you're new to backpacking, this can feel like a long way to carry all your things, especially when you're hiking on sand. Here, the sound of the ocean and of the smooth round stones shifting underfoot helps distract from the weight of your pack, which is why I love this hike as an introduction to backpacking. Once you cross Ellen Creek (which you can often see flowing into the ocean), you're allowed to set up camp. No overnight camping is permitted south of Ellen Creek. Look for markers or signs high up in the trees on the right as well; there should be a sign denoting the creek and, therefore, the start of the "campground."

Many campsites will be obvious to spot. They might sport an existing fire ring or present themselves as an obvious nook, beckoning you to nestle in between a couple of gargantuan drift logs. If one of these is open, by all means snag it. That said, you can technically camp anywhere between Ellen Creek and Hole-in-the-Wall. Make sure to pick a spot above the high-tide waterline—and know the tides. I've said it before and I'll say it again: coastal hiking requires a tide table at all times of the year. You may have to wait out the tide or hike over rocky masses protruding into the Pacific, so plan ahead and wear good shoes. The "Strip of Wilderness" brochure available at the Mora Ranger Station is full of information about the pleasures and pitfalls of coastal hiking. You'll be fine from your car to Ellen Creek, but if you continue on toward Hole-in-the-Wall, this will apply. Even if you set up camp sooner rather than later, continue on for a hike farther north along the coast. The sea stacks are beautiful to admire from a shorter distance.

Bear canisters, when not in use, should be strung up in a nearby (but not too nearby) tree. The rule of thumb is 12 feet up and 10 feet out from the nearest trunk for optimal safety. Tie a stone to the end of your rope and start tossing!

While you should always leave no trace, this is especially the place to heed that message. There aren't garbage facilities along the beach, and you'll need to pack everything out. Human waste must be buried 6–8 inches deep and 200 feet away from campsites and water sources.

Speaking of water, you can use Ellen Creek as a drinking source. Keep in mind that the tan color is normal for the coast, but you'll want to filter or boil all water no matter which stream you use. Iodine is not effective at protecting against cryptosporidium.

When I camped on the beach a couple of years ago, I had the absolute thrill of seeing a mama otter fishing for her three young pups. You'll definitely see birds and crabs and maybe some jumping fish. You could even spot whales, sea lions, or dolphins if you're very fortunate during your coastal visit. Even though this beach is not unknown by the masses, only those willing to trek their gear in will be camping here. And even with other tent campers dotting the coastline, you'll still feel like you have the whole open ocean all to yourself. Plus, the waves are excellent at muffling any neighbors' conversations.

This bears repeating: The reservations nearby are private. Be respectful.

## Rialto Beach Campground

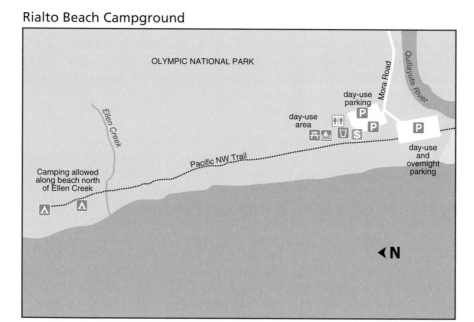

## GETTING THERE

Whether from north or south, take US 101 around the Olympic Peninsula to the town of Forks (125–200 miles from Seattle, depending on which route you take). About 1 mile north of Forks, turn west onto La Push Road/WA 110. After about 10 miles, turn right onto Mora Road, where you'll continue about 5 miles, following the signs to Rialto Beach.

**GPS COORDINATES** N47° 55.234'  W124° 38.262'

# 10

# ⚠ Upper Clearwater Campground

Beauty ★★★★ Privacy ★★★★★ Spaciousness ★★★ Quiet ★★★★★ Security ★★★ Cleanliness ★★★★★

*This refreshingly simple campground offers solitude to contrast with the overrun parts of the Olympic Peninsula.*

For sheer escapism, it's hard to beat Upper Clearwater. I'll get blasted for saying this, but there may be only one other campground on the entire Olympic Peninsula in a more remote setting that is accessible by automobile. That's Yahoo Lake, and it's right up the road from Upper Clearwater.

These Department of Natural Resources (DNR) "facilities" (it seems like a stretch to identify them as such) are for purist, minimalist tent campers. Remember minimal? OK, quick refresher: as close to a wilderness experience as possible, preferably geared more to tent camping than RVs, and scenic.

Upper Clearwater meets all three criteria—and goes no further.

Through the years, it has remained one of those best-kept secrets (allowing for the masses who will discover it through this book, of course), a place for getting the heck away from everything in a rainforest-style setting beside a river that lives up to its name.

There are six sites, all thickly shrouded in Olympic Forest vegetation, and most are on the river. Each comes with the standard-issue picnic table and fire pit with grill. Aside

Lush greens of all shades surround the secluded sites of Upper Clearwater.

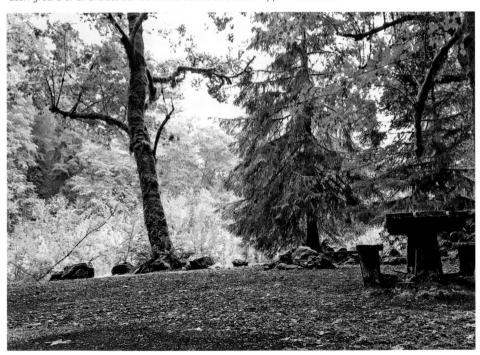

## KEY INFORMATION

**CONTACT:** 360-374-6131, dnr.wa.gov /olympicpeninsula

**OPEN:** Year-round

**SITES:** 6

**EACH SITE HAS:** Picnic table, fire pit with grill

**ASSIGNMENT:** First come, first served

**REGISTRATION:** Not necessary

**AMENITIES:** Vault toilets, nonpotable water, no garbage service, shelter, hand boat launch

**PARKING:** At individual sites

**FEE:** Free to camp; Discover Pass required to park ($11.50 per day or $35 for an annual pass)

**ELEVATION:** 900'

---

**RESTRICTIONS:**

**PETS:** On leash only

**FIRES:** In fire pits only

**ALCOHOL:** Permitted

**VEHICLES:** Small trailers only (limited side clearance)

---

from a vault toilet, the only other obvious human-made contribution is a handy shelter that could be highly desirable if you hit a particularly wet weekend. Those DNR folks think of everything!

There's also a very primitive put-in spot (for hand-carried and human-powered boats only). Frankly, at this point in the river's progress, it's difficult to imagine floating anything much larger than a rubber ducky. From its origins off an unnamed ridge just outside the Olympic National Park boundary not more than 15 miles from Upper Clearwater, the river is still fairly narrow, taking a lot of sharp turns and dropping fast while not widening much. Not until it picks up the added support of numerous feeder creeks does its flow move obviously into the river category. Keep in mind, however, that my visit was during a particularly dry late-summer weekend, so spring and early summer runoff may prove greater at higher elevations.

In fact, the Clearwater warrants mention as a decent Class I paddle stream in various books on the subject. The suggested put-in spot is at the bridge crossing (about 7 miles downriver from Upper Clearwater) with the takeout at the DNR picnic spot about 2 miles before you get to US 101. The total run is roughly 11 miles.

For higher-elevation pursuits, the area around Yahoo Lake is ripe for exploration, with hiking trails on surrounding slopes and good fishing in the lake. This is a drive-to, hike-in, end-of-road option and also a respectable camping spot (if portaging camping supplies is up your alley). Campsites are about 150 yards from the parking area (which isn't an unmanageable distance), but it's advised to put all food items or other odorous products into your car at night to avoid piquing the interest of marauding bears. This is, after all, wilderness by definition if not by designation.

It's very curious that, with all the national forest and national park lands that abound on the Olympic Peninsula, the Clearwater corridor remains in DNR hands. My impression of the DNR is that they are stewards of public lands that have not only commercial (exploitable) value but also unique characteristics deserving protection. This is an odd dichotomy, but perhaps an expected one. Speaking of this, be sure to check the Recreation Alerts on the DNR website. During my visit, a timber harvest was going on, and though I was able to drive through just fine, there can be backups on the roads. Lands on the Olympic Peninsula once fostered job security through logging and fishing, but now, with those industries floundering, they are gradually being shifted to recreational use.

As such, Upper Clearwater and its fellow DNR facilities in the area (namely Coppermine Bottom farther down the Clearwater) perhaps enjoy a more hands-off management style than the more regulated and heavily promoted facilities of the National Park Service and the U.S. Forest Service.

Enjoy it while it lasts. And thank the DNR for the ability to access a classic temperate rainforest setting, complete with old-growth specimens, in an understated fashion.

## Upper Clearwater Campground

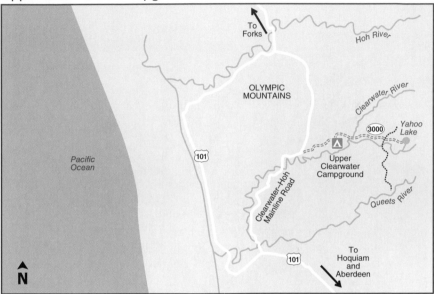

## GETTING THERE

From Queets, drive south on US 101 about 5 miles to the Clearwater–Hoh Mainline Road. Turn left, crossing the Queets River, and travel 13 paved miles to C-3000 Road. Turn right and continue 3.2 graveled, narrow miles to the campground on the right.

**GPS COORDINATES** N47° 40.735' W124° 07.102'

# PUGET
# SOUND

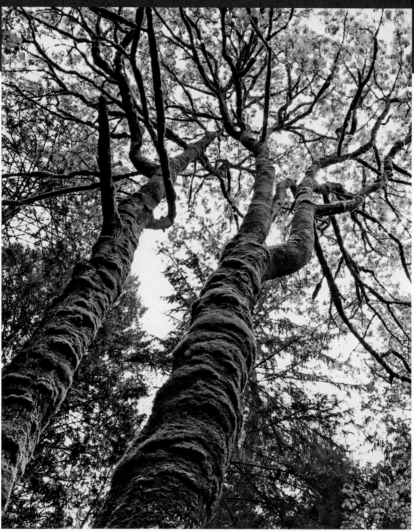

Always look up for dead branches before setting up your hammock or tent at Illahee State Park (see page 57).

# ⛺ Birch Bay State Park Campground

Beauty ★★★★★ Privacy ★★★ Spaciousness ★★★★ Quiet ★★★ Security ★★★ Cleanliness ★★★★

**This Puget Sound playground has an incredible beach and a dreamy low tide.**

It's no wonder Birch Bay is home to a number of time-shares and vacation rentals: it's a peaceful retreat on Puget Sound. It's only a couple of hours from Seattle and sits halfway between Bellingham and the US–Canada border at Peace Arch Park. Instead of spending a fortune on a peak-season vacation rental, you can reserve ahead and get a campsite at Birch Bay State Park, where you'll enjoy the same views, marvel at how far you can walk at low tide, and have the convenience of a nearby town complete with grocery stores and restaurants.

If you want to make your trip an international one, consider bringing your passport and driving across the border to explore White Rock Promenade, Campbell Valley Regional Park, Redwood Park, or the Chaberton Estate Winery. But know that you needn't travel so far to enjoy your time in nature.

Birch Bay State Park is 194 acres waiting to be explored. The bay provides 8,255 feet of saltwater shoreline and Terrell Creek has 14,923 feet of freshwater shoreline. Within the park, its several marshlands represent one of Puget Sound's only freshwater–saltwater marsh regions still intact. While the park has pockets that feel secluded, be aware that the campground is a big one.

Even on a hazy day, the mountain views at Birch Bay State Park impress.

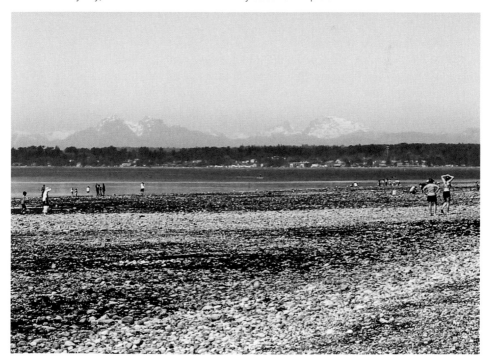

## KEY INFORMATION

**CONTACT:** 360-371-2800, Birch Bay State Park; 360-902-8844, Washington State Parks; parks.state.wa.us

**OPEN:** Year-round

**SITES:** 147 standard, 20 with water and electricity, 2 primitive, 1 group (up to 40 people), 2 group with 5 standard sites each

**EACH SITE HAS:** Picnic table, fire pit with grill, shade trees

**ASSIGNMENT:** First come, first served; reservations accepted May 15–September 15, at 888-CAMPOUT (888-226-7688) or washington.goingtocamp.com

**REGISTRATION:** Self-registration on-site, online, by phone

**AMENITIES:** Bathhouse with sinks, toilets, showers (2 ADA-compliant), hot water; firewood; boat launch nearby

**PARKING:** At individual sites

**FEE:** $25–$45 standard and utility, $12 primitive, $10 each additional vehicle

**ELEVATION:** Sea level

---

**RESTRICTIONS:**

**PETS:** On leash only

**FIRES:** In fire pits only

**ALCOHOL:** Permitted in designated sites

**VEHICLES:** Trailers and RVs up to 60' (limited availability)

---

Drive all the loops before you make a decision, especially if you're here in the off-season, when camping is first come, first served. If you enter the park from the east, you might pick a site in the forest and realize it's farther than you'd like from the water. If you make a reservation ahead of time, I like sites 17–32, or 62–74 because they're close to the water. You might prefer to be nestled in the wooded area (which can feel more private, as there's more vegetation between campsites), but I tend to want to immediately walk to the beach and spend most of my time there, gazing out at Canada or the San Juan Islands. Because there is now a convenient reservation system, reserve as far in advance as possible to secure a site at all (never mind a preferred site).

The beach draws hobbyists for oystering and clamming alike. These are public clam and oyster beaches open year-round. There's said to be good digging for a number of species, including cockles as well as Manila, littleneck, butter, and hose clams. You may want to plan ahead and pack some tools to try your hand at collecting your dinner. Don't forget to get a license—rangers check for them regularly. Be mindful of any warning signs on the beach, as a red tide can destroy the bounty for long stretches at a time. You can also check the Washington Department of Fish and Wildlife's website for Department of Health information regarding recreational shellfishing.

According to the Department of Fish and Wildlife, Birch Bay is enhanced with oyster seed. Even so, you may have slim pickings depending on the season and how many people have been out gathering. Winter oystering is one reason to head to Birch Bay in the off-season. Winter oysters are some of the most delicious.

No matter the time of year you enjoy this beachy paradise, the campground has lush amenities compared to my usual primitive suggestions. There are 8 restrooms (1 ADA-compliant) and 18 showers (2 ADA-compliant), benefits of a large, developed campground that can include more RVs than I prefer. In my mind, more campsites means more possibility for rowdy neighbors. That said, the sites are generously spaced. When I was here last June, even with many sites taken, the beach was large enough for visitors to spread out and wander off to enjoy the tidepools. And the campground seemed to be teeming with respectful tent campers. Turns out there's plenty of room for everyone! Check the tide schedule and plan your walks for when the tide is going out to have the longest window for exploration.

The beach itself compelled me to include this campground. Low tide is a marvel, even if you're not digging for clams. The horizon seems to stretch back as the tide goes out, and one feels as though one could walk forever in the space between land and ocean.

While the campground is wonderfully forested with Douglas-firs and birches and provides some pavilions for shelter, the beach does not. Be sure to bring an umbrella or pop-up canopy/tent if you're planning to lounge in the sun in the middle of summer. Some picnic tables and benches are nearby and you can sit on driftwood logs along the beach.

The road here is flat and actually has bicycle lanes. If you're yearning for antiques shops, a candy store, and a cute town experience to round out your camping adventure, riding a bicycle north from Birch Bay is a nice way to explore. Whatever brought you to this northern stretch of Puget Sound, you're bound to enjoy yourself—and the sunset.

## GETTING THERE

From Bellingham, take I-5 North, and get off at Exit 266. Turn left onto Grandview Road. In about 6 miles, continue through a roundabout to stay on Grandview. In a mile, turn right onto Jackson Road. A mile after that, turn left onto Helweg Road, and you'll be entering the park from the east side. Note that from the town of Birch Bay, you can approach the park on the northwest side, via Birch Bay Road.

**GPS COORDINATES** N48° 54.204' W122° 45.941'

## Birch Bay State Park Campground

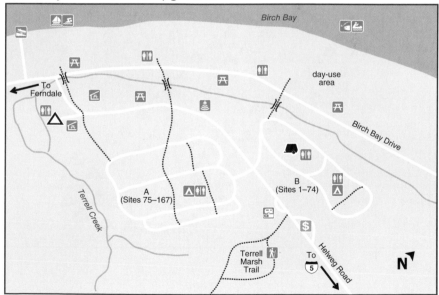

*See next page for detail maps of Loops A and B.*

## Loop A

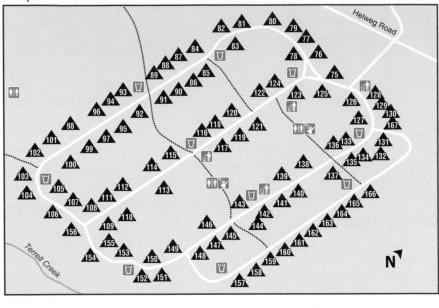

## Loop B

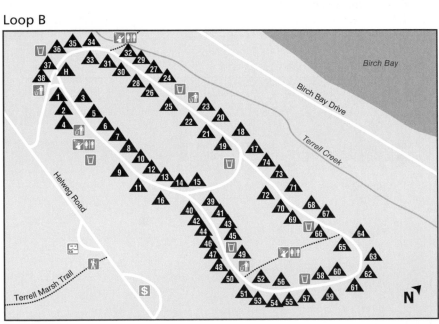

# 12

# Deception Pass State Park:
## BOWMAN BAY CAMPGROUND

Beauty ★★★★★ Privacy ★★★ Spaciousness ★★★ Quiet ★★★★ Security ★★★ Cleanliness ★★★★★

*Located in the less overrun part of Deception Pass State Park, this campground is tucked away in a saltwater bayside setting with historical significance.*

Washington's state parks are seldom escapes from the crowds, and Deception Pass State Park is no exception. They are, however, almost always delightful escapes from the ordinary, and Deception Pass reigns supreme in this department.

Anchored on both sides of the body of water that separates Whidbey Island from Fidalgo Island, Deception Pass State Park literally offers something for everybody—even tent campers. Although believing that you might find yourself alone at any point during the summer season is insane, this area is so appealing that, in deference to the tent-camping mandate of this book, I must include it. I gave serious thought to nixing it when I visited the park several times during the summer of 2004, but it's too spectacular! I can't help it if lots of other people think so too.

However, a portion of the park seems to be largely overlooked. It could be the signage (or lack thereof) that causes a problem. (Whatever it is, I'm not tellin' when I find out!)

First, the section of campsites on the north side of the park (the Fidalgo Island side) number only 20 (compared with 230 in the Whidbey Island sector). Don't be confused by the fact that they are numbered 271–290 and are reservable. (I highly recommend a reservation if you can plan ahead a few months during the peak season.)

Bowman Bay is the smallest campground in Deception Pass State Park (not counting the boat-in-only campgrounds).

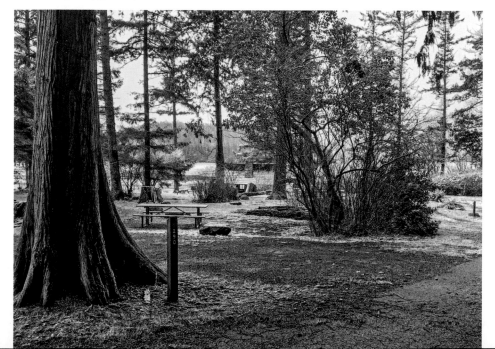

**CONTACT:** 360-902-8844, parks.state.wa.us

**OPEN:** Facility year-round, campsites closed in winter

**SITES:** 16 sites (2 with hookups)

**EACH SITE HAS:** Picnic table, fire pit with grill

**ASSIGNMENT:** First come, first served, or by reservation at 888-CAMPOUT (888-226-7688) or parks.state.wa.us; reservations recommended during peak season; reservations accepted up to 9 months in advance

**REGISTRATION:** On site, online, and by phone

**AMENITIES:** ADA-compliant restrooms with showers, group shelter with tables and cooking space, picnic area, historical interpretive center, boat launch, fishing pier

**PARKING:** At individual sites

**FEE:** $25, $10 each additional vehicle

**ELEVATION:** Sea level

---

**RESTRICTIONS:**

**PETS:** On leash only

**FIRES:** In fire pits only, wood gathering prohibited

**ALCOHOL:** In designated areas

**VEHICLES:** Trailers and RVs 18–35', some sites limited to 18'

Second, the sites themselves are obviously geared toward tent camping. The camp road is narrow, it follows the somewhat hilly contour of the bulk of Rosario Head on which it sits, the parking spurs are tight, there are no hookups, and the sites are decently spaced, with generous undergrowth between each. The general sense of the place is one of intimate and uncluttered relaxation in a very natural state—the absence of RVs (with the exception of the camp host parked at the outermost space on the outbound end of the loop) helps. Compare this to the crush of campsites with pull-throughs and hookups over on Whidbey Island, and you'll be back here in a flash.

The geography further promotes this sector of the park as the domain of tent campers and a more simplified—dare I say more dignified?—park experience. Bowman Bay's silky, protected waters within the curve of the shoreline glisten before you. Views of headlands covered with weather-beaten madrones and evergreens contrast directly with the sandy shoreline at your feet. A former bathhouse built by the Civilian Conservation Corps back in the 1930s has been restored and serves as an interpretive center, lending its own timeworn quality to the scene. Tucked into the hillside above the camp road, the ranger's quaint quarters complete the picture-perfect setting.

A look at the statistics of this magnificent park will quickly lead you to conclude that exploring its sprawling environs is a must—which is best done by foot, bike, or boat. For starters, the park encompasses 4,134 acres. There are 38 miles of hiking trails, 77,000 feet of saltwater frontage, and 33,900 feet of fresh water divided among four lakes. Boats have 710 feet of saltwater dock access, 1,980 feet of saltwater moorage, and 450 feet of freshwater dock access. There are wetlands, sand dunes, interpretive trails, historical monuments—including the Maiden of Deception Pass, which depicts the story of Ko-Kwal-alwoot of the Samish Indian Nation—a saltwater fishing pier, and an astonishing array of wildlife, sea life, and birds. If that's not enough to keep you busy for at least a week of vacation, sit in on a weekend ranger program at one of the two amphitheaters and see what you missed.

For all that Deception Pass State Park has to offer, I feel compelled to lodge one small complaint. The bridge that connects the parts of this remarkable area is an engineering marvel, and the views from it are unequalled, but I have never understood the logic behind allowing pedestrians to wander along what is often a windswept or fogbound catwalk with major traffic whizzing by. Gives me the willies!

## Deception Pass State Park: Bowman Bay Campground

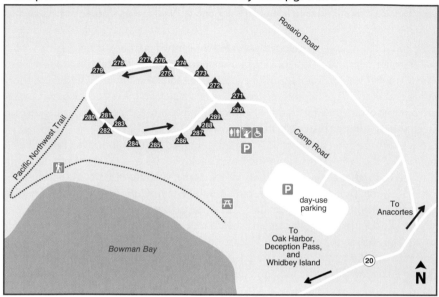

## GETTING THERE

From Anacortes, drive 9 miles south on WA 20. Turn right onto Rosario Road, then make an immediate left (and I mean immediate) onto the camp access road at the sign for Bowman Bay. Drive down the cool, forested lane, and continue straight beyond the sign for the boat launch to the camping loop.

**GPS COORDINATES** N48° 25.013'  W122° 38.721'

# 13

# Fort Ebey State Park Campground

Beauty ★★★★ Privacy ★★★ Spaciousness ★★★★ Quiet ★★★ Security ★★★★★ Cleanliness ★★★★

*Hop a ferry—preferably the one that leaves from Mukilteo, south of Everett—and head for the westernmost tip of Whidbey Island to enjoy one of Washington's newest state parks.*

Situated in blissfully underdeveloped waterfront beauty, Fort Ebey is increasingly popular among tent campers and others looking to escape urban life without having to travel too far.

The fort itself was one of four artillery facilities established in 1942 to defend the state during World War II. The other three forts (Casey, Flagler, and Worden) also occupy choice waterfront real estate on either side of Admiralty Inlet, joining Ebey in guarding the mouth of Puget Sound today as historic state parks.

From a tent-camping perspective, Fort Ebey—named for the pioneering Isaac Ebey family that settled the area—is decidedly the least developed. It's evident that every attempt has been made to protect the natural beauty of the place. Old-growth Douglas-fir marks this region, which escaped desecration by logging interests. An undergrowth of salal, huckleberry, Scotch broom, and rhododendron has become quite dense over the years, making each campsite decidedly singular and private. In mid-spring the wild rhododendrons fill the park with a profusion of large, colorful blossoms.

The tent area is to the left as you pass the campground office; beach access, picnic areas, and Lake Pondilla are to the right. On the way to the campground is the turnoff to the

Fort Ebey's walk-in sites are worth strolling past, even if they're full when you arrive.

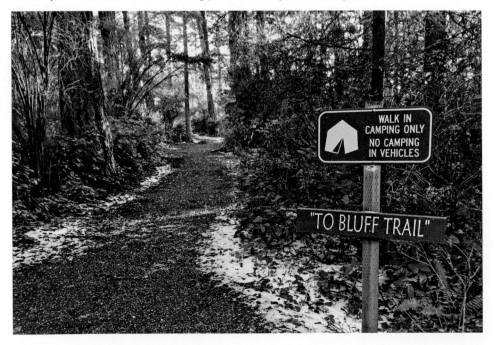

## KEY INFORMATION

**CONTACT:** 360-678-4636, Fort Ebey State Park; 360-902-8844, Washington State Parks; parks.state.wa.us

**OPEN:** February 28–October 31

**SITES:** 39 standard, 11 with electric and water hookups, 1 group (up to 60 people), 1 nonreservable marine trail

**EACH SITE HAS:** Picnic table, fire pit with grill, shade trees

**ASSIGNMENT:** First come, first served; reservations accepted May 15–September 15, at 888-CAMPOUT (888-226-7688)

**REGISTRATION:** At campground office

**AMENITIES:** Bathhouse with sinks, toilets, showers, hot water; public telephone; picnic area; group camp; boat put-in

**PARKING:** At individual sites

**FEE:** Varies depending on site and season: $20–$37 standard, $25–$45 partial hookup with either electric or water, $30–$50 full hookup, $12 marine trail, $154.98 group camp

**ELEVATION:** Sea level

**RESTRICTIONS:**

**PETS:** On leash only

**FIRES:** In fire pits only, wood gathering prohibited

**ALCOHOL:** Permitted

**VEHICLES:** Trailers and RVs up to 32' at some sites; up to 30 vehicles at group site (of those, up to 2 can be RVs that are 18' or less, and up to 20 can be RVs or trailers that are 10' or less)

old gun emplacements that have long since been dismantled but continue to instill—even if only momentarily—the sense of vulnerability that prevailed during World War II, when one looked out over the wide expanse of the Strait of Juan de Fuca and the Pacific Ocean.

Continuing on to the campground, enter the loop to the right and know that you're passing the best sites early on. If they're empty, grab one. These are pull-throughs but without hookups, so don't feel guilty if your compact car looks a little lost in the parking space. These premier bluffside sites have short trail access to the wild, windward side of Whidbey Island. You'll have your own endless view and a sharp taste of the elements if the wind is blowing (chances are good).

This area of western Washington tends to be less rainy than other parts (although nearly every time I've been there, it's been blustery and wet) because it's protected by the rain shadow cast by the Olympic Mountains to the west. This said, the weather manages to wreak havoc on the place in other ways. It may be drier at Fort Ebey, but it's not necessarily tamer. The park faces the Strait of Juan de Fuca and is constantly buffeted by Pacific winds.

The delicate composition of glacial debris—sand and gravel—that makes up Whidbey Island is often no match for the howling furies that descend. Point Partridge, which I remember as a high, grassy bluff, has been gnawed and clawed beyond recognition by the vengeance of seasonal storms. More than 2,000 of the majestic old-growth firs that once graced the park grounds toppled like matchsticks in the fierce snow and windstorm of December 1990, and a second storm in the late 1990s added insult to injury. Cleanup teams struggled for many years to deal with the downed giants.

There are plenty of activities within the 645-acre park: beachcombing along the driftwood-laden shoreline; hiking the wooded trails along the bluffline; fishing for bass in freshwater Lake Pondilla; watching a surprising variety of wildlife, including bald eagles, deer, geese, ducks, raccoons, rabbits, pheasants, and grouse; and seeking out the varieties of cactus (yes, cactus!) that grow in this unusual banana-belt region of western Washington.

If none of this satisfies you, numerous attractions in Coupeville and Oak Harbor may fill in the gaps. Several other state parks are in the neighborhood too. Of particular note is Fort Casey, which has an interpretive center and is the site of Admiralty Head Lighthouse. Ebey's Landing National Historic Reserve preserves the legacy of the early pioneers.

It's worth noting that the park attendants have been known to turn away as many as 200 cars per day during heavy summer usage. This park takes reservations in the summertime, so either plan far enough ahead or consider the splendor of the off-season (but avoid the hurricane-force winds).

If this is your first time to Fort Ebey State Park, you should know that although signs mark the way to the campground, you will drive through a light residential area. It may not seem that there is a park nearby, but keep going.

## Fort Ebey State Park Campground

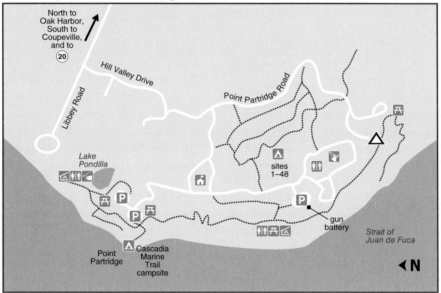

## GETTING THERE

From Seattle, drive north on I-5 and WA 525/526 to Mukilteo and the Washington State Ferry terminal for Whidbey Island. Once on the island, follow WA 525 north, pick up WA 20 at Keystone; continue north to Libbey Road and follow the signs to the park. Total driving distance on the island is about 35 miles.

ALTERNATE ROUTE: From I-5 at Burlington, take WA 20 west and drive down the northern half of Whidbey Island through Deception Pass. Look for Libbey Road and the park turnoff to the right, about 8 miles south of Oak Harbor, not long after Penn Cove.

GPS COORDINATES  N48° 13.487'  W122° 46.130'

# 14

# Illahee State Park Campground

Beauty ★★★★ Privacy ★★★★ Spaciousness ★★★★ Quiet ★★★★ Security ★★★★ Cleanliness ★★★★★

*Undiscovered yet convenient, this lovely place is for those who don't feel like taking an endless drive to get away from it all.*

Here is one of those classic Northwest spots that makes spontaneous car camping such a delightful proposition in this region.

Situated on a high bluff that guards the southern entrance to Port Orchard passage, Illahee State Park is a gem of a destination roughly an hour west of Seattle by ferry and about half that amount of time by car from Tacoma. Or you can get here on the Edmonds–Kingston ferry (just north of Seattle) and sightsee your way south with numerous side trips. With 1,785 feet of saltwater frontage on the bay and a 354-foot dock with a flotilla of moorage buoys, you could easily slip into this quiet haven by boat.

The park faces northeast, out of the way on the northern outskirts of Bremerton and overlooking the west side of Bainbridge Island. Until it was acknowledged as a most livable city on a national magazine's top-ten list, Bremerton was known to the outside world mostly as a ship-building port and home to the navy's Pacific Fleet. Since then, it hasn't exactly attracted the rich and famous, but when Seattle's housing market went through the roof a few years back and freeway traffic jams reached road-rage proportions, West Sound communities started heavily promoting their affordable housing, stress-free ferry riding, and general quality of life.

Illahee State Park is full of beautiful old-growth trees (400-year-old yew not pictured).

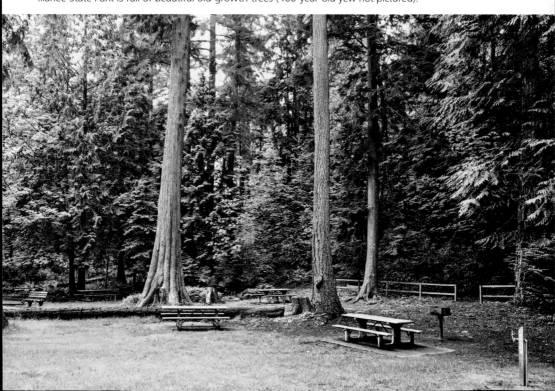

## KEY INFORMATION

**CONTACT:** 360-478-6460, Illahee State Park; 360-902-8844, Washington State Parks; parks.state.wa.us

**OPEN:** Year-round

**SITES:** 23 standard, 2 full hookup, 5 hiker/biker

**EACH SITE HAS:** Picnic table, fire pit with grill, shade trees

**ASSIGNMENT:** First come, first served; reservations accepted May 15–September 15 at 888-CAMPOUT (226-7688) and washington.goingtocamp.com

**REGISTRATION:** Self-registration on-site, online, or by phone

**AMENITIES:** Restrooms with toilets, sinks, hot showers, 2 ADA-compliant; boat launch, mooring buoys, boat dock; public telephone; trailer dump station; horseshoe pits, ballfield, playground; group picnic areas with covered kitchens

**PARKING:** At individual sites and in parking lot at shoreline

**FEE:** $25–$45 standard and utility, $12 hiker/biker, $10 each additional vehicle

**ELEVATION:** 295'

---

**RESTRICTIONS:**

**PETS:** On leash only

**FIRES:** In fire pits only

**ALCOHOL:** Permitted in designated areas

**VEHICLES:** RVs up to 32', no hookups at standard sites

Illahee (a Native American word meaning "earth" or "country") is prime real estate supporting the lifestyle to which West Sounders subscribe. It still appears to be unknown to most out-of-towners (too busy searching for their own affordable "illahee," I guess), which is good news for the rest of us. Amid towering and densely clustered maples, cedars, Douglas-firs, madrones, dogwoods, and rhododendrons, each campsite is picturesquely and privately shrouded in ferns, salals, huckleberries, blackberries (watch out for the thorns), and salmonberries.

William Bremer, for whom Bremerton is named, first settled in the area around 1888, salivating at the abundant timber resources. Fortunately, he set to work clearing other areas first, and Illahee was spared the ax and chainsaw. The state acquired the area in seven separate parcels, beginning in 1934; much of the original foliage has been left intact. In fact, Illahee State Park is home to the only remaining stand of old-growth forest in Kitsap County and one of the largest yew trees in the country. This alone makes a visit worth the trip.

After setting up camp and with the sound of seagulls screeching overhead, take one of the park trails leading down to the waterfront. The drop is steep, so you'll get a good start on your exercise program. There is a paved roadway down to the water as well, but it's sharply inclined and narrow with no room for pedestrians—nowhere to go if you happen to meet up with an SUV–boat trailer combination on any of the several blind, hairpin turns along the way. So I advise the path if you intend to walk.

Park developers got a little carried away with the size of the parking lot down on the beach, but in all likelihood the lot was intended to accommodate the many boaters using the launch on busy summer weekends. It's a prime spot to put in and explore the shorelines along Puget Sound. Sea kayaking from this spot is an excellent idea because you can explore the myriad coves, inlets, bays, hooks, points, and passages that define the land.

There's plenty of marine life and the usual assortment of camp critters on shore (squirrels, chipmunks, and raccoons) to observe. At low tide, clamming can be quite good. Crabbing and oystering are options, but first check that there are no restrictions. Red tide and pollution indiscriminately plague beaches around Puget Sound. Generally, there will be signs warning of any current hazards.

The park honors more than just old-growth trees. A veteran's war memorial pays tribute to local fallen heroes, which may help explain the giant gun that sits guarding the entrance to the park (not your typical welcoming attraction at a campground). Other points of interest in the surrounding area include the quaint Scandinavian town of Poulsbo, the Suquamish Museum as well as the town of Suquamish, Port Orchard's antiques malls, the Navy's Trident submarine base in Bangor, and the Hood Canal Brewery near Kingston. A number of first-class golf courses are within a short drive of the campground.

## Illahee State Park Campground

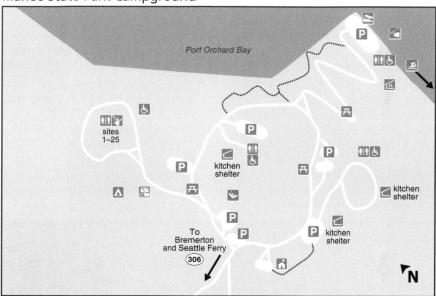

## GETTING THERE

From the Bremerton Ferry Terminal, follow WA 303 north (Warren Avenue) to WA 306 (Sylvan Way). Turn right and follow the signs to Illahee. The total distance is about 3 miles.

From Tacoma, cross the Tacoma Narrows Bridge on WA 16 and follow the road (it merges with WA 3 in Gorst) about 25 miles to Bremerton. Take the City Center exit (WA 304), which zigzags through town. Keep making the obvious zigzags until you reach WA 303 (Warren Avenue). Turn left and continue to WA 306 (Sylvan Way). Turn right and follow the signs to Illahee.

**GPS COORDINATES** N47° 35.738' W122° 35.788'

# 15

# ⚠ Larrabee State Park Campground

Beauty ★★★★ Privacy ★★★ Spaciousness ★★★★ Quiet ★★★ Security ★★★ Cleanliness ★★★★★

*Only 7 miles from Bellingham, this park will give you a respectable nature fix when you're on a tight schedule.*

Camping within 7 miles of an urban center doesn't qualify as a true wilderness escape. But when time, inclination, or myriad other factors don't allow you to throw yourself into a far-flung adventure, the unspoiled pleasure of Larrabee State Park can be quite a decent substitute. To be honest, I thought of cutting this campground, but the beauty of the beach simply would not allow it.

Located on 2,683 acres along saltwater Samish Bay south of Bellingham, Larrabee is the oldest state park in Washington. Its designation in 1915 was a mere 20 acres. But with acquisitions and contributions over the years, the park has been able to protect such a lush growth of Northwest foliage—Douglas-firs, western red cedars, hemlocks, big-leaf maples, willows, rhododendrons, and sword ferns—that it is difficult not to think you have ventured miles into a remote and primeval place.

In reality, the way to Larrabee is along one of the most heavily traveled scenic drives in western Washington and perhaps the entire state. Chuckanut Drive is officially known as

Perhaps take a moment (or a few hours) to sit on the rocks at Larrabee State Park and gaze across Bellingham Bay toward Lummi Island.

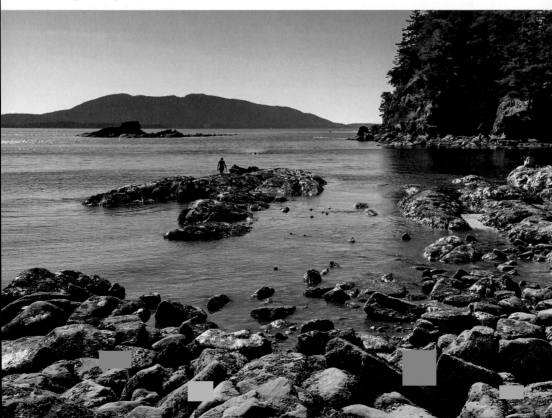

## KEY INFORMATION

**CONTACT:** 360-676-2093, Larrabee State Park; 360-902-8844, Washington State Parks; parks.state.wa.us

**OPEN:** Year-round

**SITES:** 51 standard, 26 with utilities, 8 primitive

**EACH SITE HAS:** Picnic table, fire pit with grill, shade trees

**ASSIGNMENT:** First come, first served; reservations accepted May 15–September 15, at 888-CAMPOUT (888-226-7688) or washington.goingtocamp.com

**REGISTRATION:** Self-registration on-site, online, by phone

**AMENITIES:** Bathhouse with sinks, toilets, showers (4 ADA-compliant), hot water; boat launch nearby

**PARKING:** At individual sites or in campground lot

**FEE:** $25–$45 standard and utility, $12 primitive, $10 each additional vehicle

**ELEVATION:** Sea level to 1,100'

---

**RESTRICTIONS:**

**PETS:** On leash only

**FIRES:** In fire pits only

**ALCOHOL:** Permitted in designated areas

**VEHICLES:** Maximum site length is 60' (limited availability)

WA 11 and connects south Bellingham with the farming communities of the Skagit River flats along 25 miles of roadway with numerous stretches that cling precariously to the side of Chuckanut Mountain. A series of wheel-gripping twists and turns eventually gives way to a straightaway that makes you accelerate just for the sheer joy of seeing broad, flat ground all around you.

Chuckanut Drive is famous not only for its suicide turns but also for the stupendous views across Puget Sound to the San Juan Archipelago. Scenic overlook turnouts allow you to pause and take a more leisurely gape, not to mention get that string of Mario Andretti wannabes off your tail. A couple of first-rate seafood restaurants along Chuckanut also make the drive a popular outing, but if you're too busy watching the brake lights of the car in front of you, you might miss them the first time through.

For reasons that defy explanation, Chuckanut Drive attracts a sizable number of cyclists. I don't recommend it myself simply because it's too dangerous. The road is very narrow, with blind corners, minimal shoulders, and too many lurching RVs and impatient SUVs for my taste. Aside from an occasional turnout, there is no place to go to avoid or be avoided, short of slamming into the crumbling rock of Chuckanut Mountain or careening over a guardrail into space. The BIKE ROUTE marker should have some fine print on it.

So leave the bicycle at home on this trip. You have plenty of hiking trails, pebbled beaches, and rocky tidepools to explore instead. Sea kayaking is also an option, with numerous coves, bays, rocks, and islets within easy paddling range. For boaters or saltwater-fishing types, a boat launch is nearby. For freshwater anglers, both Fragrance Lake and Lost Lake are stocked, but they require a little effort to get to (along a 2-mile trail). Bird-watching, swimming, and scuba diving have their seasonal appeal.

If you simply want fresh air and a look at the lay of the land, take a drive up Cleator Road to 1,900-foot Cyrus Gates Overlook for the best possible view of the San Juans. For views of Mount Baker (Washington's third-highest volcano, only 30 miles east) and the North Cascade Range, take the short hike to East Overlook.

Weather-wise, this is coastal Washington, so let's be realistic. Westerly winds carry moisture and cool temperatures most of the year, with late summer and early fall the most dependable times for dry tenting. Even on the hottest summer days, marine breezes chill the skin, and it's a rare evening that doesn't warrant a fleece layer. Summer evenings this close to the US–Canada border last a long time; it's not uncommon for the last strains of a fabulous sunset to be visible after 11 p.m.

You'll find the campground to the right as you descend the camp road off Chuckanut Drive. Two small loops flank the entrance to the camping area and feature individual and multiple standard sites. Two larger loops offer standard individual and multiple sites on their perimeter, with the utility sites smartly clustered within. Sites 1–29 are close to Chuckanut Drive (above you), so, if possible, try for sites 34–41. Sites 42–46 are tucked among bushy thickets and seemingly private, but keep in mind that railroad tracks are just south, and numerous trains (including Amtrak) rumble by day and night. The walk-in sites are probably the best option for both privacy and quiet, but they're not reservable and can easily fill on any given summer weekend. If you can plan ahead for one of the standard sites, do. Reservations should be made as far in advance as possible.

## Larrabee State Park Campground

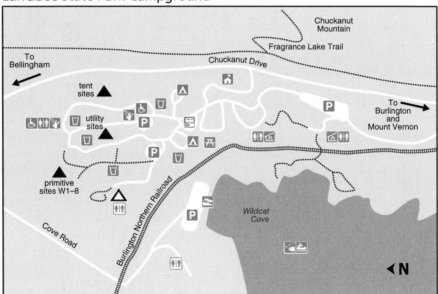

## GETTING THERE

From Seattle, drive north on I-5 to Bellingham and take the turnoff for Chuckanut Drive and Fairhaven. Follow the signs to WA 11 and head south on WA 11/Chuckanut Drive. The entrance to the park is about 7 miles on the right.

**GPS COORDINATES** N48° 39.187' W122° 29.408'

# 16

# Lopez Farm Cottages and Tent Camping

Beauty ★★★★ Privacy ★★★★★ Spaciousness ★★★★★ Quiet ★★★ Security ★★★★★ Cleanliness ★★★★★

*This is camping for adults in an indulgent and thoughtfully designed private preserve.*

You'll notice that this book and its companion, *Best Tent Camping: Oregon,* are mostly collections of camping spots run by public agencies (national parks, state parks, national forests, Department of Natural Resources, and so on). I try to stay away from private operations because they usually do not meet my camping criteria, are almost always monopolized by RVs, and aren't exactly places where you can count on respectful camp neighbors. The health of a private campground is also directly dependent on the owner's ability to run it in the black, and it often reflects a tight operating budget and a make-do mentality (not unlike a lot of landlords I've known in my time).

Every once in a while, along comes an exception to the rule. Lopez Farm Cottages and Tent Camping easily qualifies as a worthwhile destination for blending this island's most-needed services (thoughtful tent camping and private cottages) tastefully and practically. If you plan to bring the kids, however, think again. Lopez Farm accommodates no one under

The camp building, where a light snow had fallen the morning I ferried in to visit

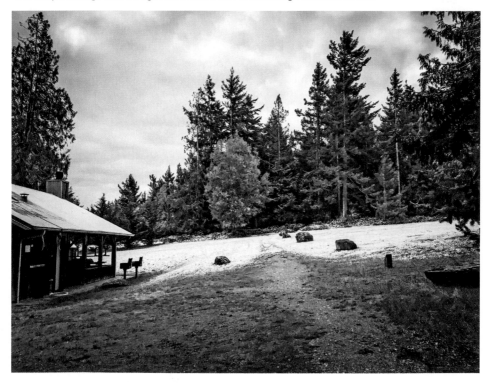

## KEY INFORMATION

**CONTACT:** 360-468-3555, lopezfarm
cottages.com

**OPEN:** Memorial Day–September 30, with
sites A, B, C open only July 1–Labor Day

**SITES:** 12 for tents; 3 for cars, camper vans,
or trucks with camper shells; 2 camp nests
(which include a queen-sized futon with
bedding, carpeting, and ice chests)

**EACH SITE HAS:** Level tent area, hammock,
2 Adirondack chairs, small table

**ASSIGNMENT:** First come, first served, or by
reservation at lopezfarmcottages.com

**REGISTRATION:** Self-registration on-site
and online

**AMENITIES:** Wooded setting, camp building
with private bathrooms and open-air hot
showers, picnic tables, badminton net,
barbecues, complimentary morning coffee,
wagons for moving camping equipment

**PARKING:** In separate area near the
check-in building

**FEE:** $48–$52 per site, double occupancy;
$10 each additional person (maximum 4
per site); $88–$98 camp nest (depending
on the month)

**ELEVATION:** 170'

---

### RESTRICTIONS:

**PETS:** No pets (unless you're staying in
cottage 4)

**FIRES:** Open fires at campsites prohibited,
hibachis and campstoves are OK

**ALCOHOL:** Permitted

**VEHICLES:** Trailers and RVs not permitted

**OTHER:** No children under age 14

---

the age of 14 (except for an adorable assortment of the four-legged variety—mostly lambs, fawns, and baby rabbits).

Just minutes from the Lopez Island ferry terminal and only 1 mile from the village of Lopez, Lopez Farm is picturesque—situated in the middle of a broad, rolling meadow defined on three sides by the Lopez Island road system and on one side by forest. Now, you might protest that a campground described as bounded on three sides by roadway can't possibly offer pastoral quiet, but the compound is laid out so expertly that this is a minor consideration.

And if you know anything about the roads on Lopez (besides that everyone waves), then you know they are busiest when ferries are arriving and departing, which is only a temporary intrusion—and not a very late one at that! Ferries between the mainland ferry terminal at Anacortes, Lopez (the first stop), and the rest of the islands don't offer service much after 9 p.m. on weekdays (about an hour or so later on Fridays and Saturdays). It's important to know the ferry schedule intimately when traveling in the San Juan Islands, by the way.

The main campground will be on your left as you drive in from Fisherman Bay Road. Follow the road as it curls around to the right, however. At the fork, stay right for campsites 1–10; bear left for sites A, B, and C. Find your designated parking area, sign in at the check-in building, and pick up a handy wagon for transporting your camping gear. Since campsites are available on a first-come, first-served basis (if you haven't reserved your first night in advance by credit card), you'll want to take a look at the sites before you choose. Sites A, B, and C are used as group sites and are available individually if sites 1–10 are taken.

Some of the sites in the main camping area have the advantage of being closer to the camp building's amenities, whereas those at the far end of the loop offer maximum privacy. Each has its own "personality" and all come with effects that will remind you of your backyard—hammock, Adirondack chairs, and a small table. If I had to pick the optimum spot for my tastes, I would have to say it's site 9, which mixes all the characteristics that will spoil you for camping at Lopez Farm: an easy stroll to the Scandinavian-style camp building, views of sheep resting among the old apple trees, and maybe just a tad more isolation, thanks to a dense cluster of foliage. It's hard to beat the bucolic ambience of a Lopez Farm tent-camping experience.

Central to the experience is the camp building—a cleverly designed multiuse facility with lots of natural wood; a giant, covered stone fireplace at one end; and four private bathrooms (two with dual-showerhead showers) at the other. There are picnic tables both inside and out, barbecues beside the camp building, and even a microwave. Morning coffee (how much more civilized can you get?) will be waiting for you on the pasture side of the camp building. Since open fires are not allowed at the campsites, the fireplace will be the main attraction at night. In a storm, it's easy to imagine the roaring blaze kicking off an unplanned get-acquainted session among fellow campers—maybe even the spark of a romance.

The campground is open only from May to October, but if you find yourself in Lopez in the off-season, Lopez Farm has five comfortably appointed cottages available by reservation all year long. Whether it's camping or cottaging, a visit to Lopez Farm is a definite dose of indulgence. And you're worth it!

## Lopez Farm Cottages and Tent Camping

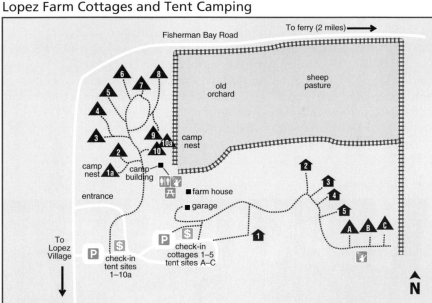

## GETTING THERE

From the ferry terminal at Lopez Island in the San Juans, drive 2.6 miles inland toward Lopez Village. The driveway and well-placed sign will be on your left. The entrance is the first driveway you come to; the exit is the second. Follow the signs to either the CAMPING check-in building for sites 1–10 or the COTTAGE check-in building for sites A, B, and C.

**GPS COORDINATES** N48° 32.433' W122° 54.272'

# 17

# Moran State Park:
## MOUNTAIN LAKE CAMPGROUND

Beauty ★★★★ Privacy ★★★★ Spaciousness ★★★★ Quiet ★★★★★ Security ★★★★ Cleanliness ★★★★★

*Moran State Park is the crowning glory of the San Juan Islands. Mount Constitution offers views of the Olympic Mountains to the south, the Cascades to the east, the Canadian Rockies to the north, and a 360-degree view of the islands that stud Puget Sound.*

A 5,252-acre preserve featuring primarily old-growth forest, Moran State Park has 30 miles of hiking trails, 25 miles of biking trails (restricted in the summer to 11 miles), and 6 miles of riding trails. It encompasses several lakes, numerous streams, and two iconic waterfalls. Mount Constitution, at 2,409 feet, is the highest point in the San Juan Islands, offering panoramic views said to be among the world's best. On a clear day, you can see the Olympic Mountains, the Cascades, the Canadian Rockies, Mount Baker, Mount Rainier, the lakes of Moran State Park, and a 360-degree view of Puget Sound. Plus, there's a stone observation tower to enhance the view.

The park as a whole has 151 tent sites, 1 dump station, 5 restrooms (1 of which is ADA-compliant), and 10 showers (2 of which are ADA-compliant). There are boat launches on Cascade Lake and Mountain Lake, and use is restricted to nonmotorized craft.

The main facilities at Cascade Lake are overcrowded and close to a road, but if you go a mile farther, to Mountain Lake, you will find one of the best campgrounds in Washington. Mountain Lake is a quiet set of 10 tent sites and 1 group site situated in two loops on the shore of a quiet, often glass-smooth lake. The water reflects the old-growth trees back at the sky, and it's easy to forget that you arrived by car.

The lake is circled by an easy, flat trail about 4 miles long that runs through the forest and past a dam with pleasant views. The path intersects with trails to Cascade Lake, Cascade Falls,

A site with a water view

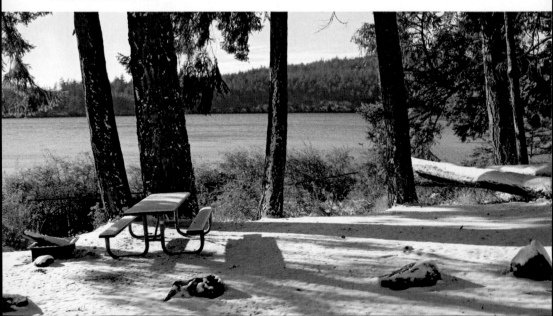

## KEY INFORMATION

**CONTACT:** 360-376-2326, Moran State Park; 360-902-8844, Washington State Parks; parks.state.wa.us

**OPEN:** Year-round, parts of the park closed in winter

**SITES:** 10 standard, 1 group (up to 60 people)

**EACH SITE HAS:** Fire pit

**ASSIGNMENT:** First come, first served; reservations accepted May 15–September 15, at 888-CAMPOUT (888-226-7688) or washington.goingtocamp.com; reservations not required but recommended; $8 fee for online reservations

**REGISTRATION:** At ranger station on Olga Road (near entrance to park), online, and by phone

**AMENITIES:** Vault toilets, potable water, walking distance to comfort station, which is open in the summer (1 in camp and 1 at group camp)

**PARKING:** Up to 2 vehicles at individual sites

**FEE:** $25–$35 standard, $30–$45 with utilities, $12 primitive, $10 each additional vehicle, $156.34 for group site (up to 60 people)

**ELEVATION:** 1,100'

---

**RESTRICTIONS:**

**PETS:** On leash only, prohibited on swimming beaches

**QUIET HOURS:** 10 p.m.–6:30 a.m.

**FIRES:** In grated pits only

**VEHICLES:** Maximum 2 cars per site, no more than 4 people per car; trailers up to 18'

**ALCOHOL:** Permitted

Twin Lakes, and Mount Constitution, all of which are well worth a visit. Stop among the old-growth cedars and watch a kingfisher watch the water. Listen to him cackle across the lake, as wild and lonely as a loon, and see him dip into the water and come up with a trout.

Sites at Mountain Lake book quickly. Reservations are necessary, and you may need to make them well in advance of a trip. On top of that, it's a fairly expensive campground. There are a few primitive sites along the road to Mount Constitution that cost less, but they're away from attractions and close to the road.

Mountain Lake is an ideal place for a quiet hiking retreat. With several options for day hiking directly from your campsite, you won't even have to get in your car. The Mountain Lake loop is 4 miles long and circles the deep, still surface of Mountain Lake with views of the water most of the way. Walk an extra 3 miles for a loop of Twin Lakes, a pair of still ponds with no one around. Other interesting hikes include either of the Mount Constitution trails, one that passes Twin Lakes and another that offers access to Summit Lake; Mount Pickett Trail; Cascade Lake Trail; Cascade Creek Trail; and Cascade Falls Trail.

Watch for black-tailed or mule deer (some of which are white), minks, otters, ospreys, hawks, eagles, herons, hummingbirds, geese, grouse, owls, and swans. The lake is full of bass and rainbow, cutthroat, and kokanee trout. Please read catch restrictions before fishing.

Visit Moran for days of quiet hikes and stunning views. Paddle on the lakes and explore the island. See the old growth, the seed logs, the mosses and ferns. Watch the salmon swim upstream. Moran is a beautiful park, and Mountain Lake is centrally located, ideally situated for exploring what it has to offer.

## GETTING THERE

Take the Washington State Ferry from Anacortes, WA, or Sidney, BC, to Orcas Island. Follow the signs to Eastsound, about 8 miles, and turn right onto Main Street, traveling through town as it becomes Crescent Beach Drive. After about 1 mile, turn right onto Olga Road. Follow the signs to Moran State Park. Just past Cascade Lake, turn left and follow the signs toward Mount Constitution. After 1 mile, a clearly marked sign for Mountain Lake is on the right. The parking lot is a quarter mile farther, the campsites just past that.

**GPS COORDINATES** N48° 39.400' W122° 49.085'

## Moran State Park Campgrounds

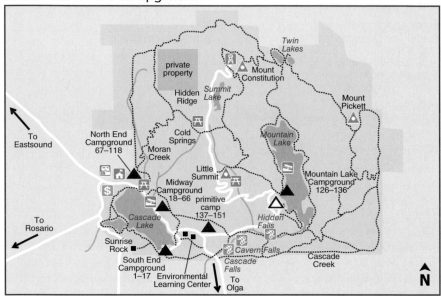

## Mountain Lake Campground

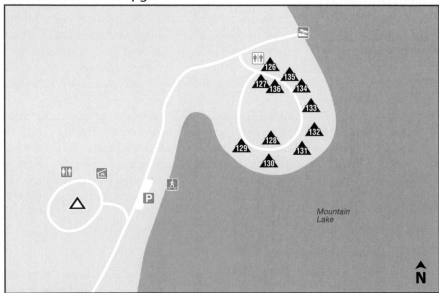

# 18

# Obstruction Pass State Park Campground

Beauty ★★★★★ Privacy ★★★★ Spaciousness ★★★★ Quiet ★★★★ Security ★★★★★ Cleanliness ★★★★★

*With water views, lush old-growth forest, and an array of wildlife, this is a place of quiet beauty and simple pleasures.*

Obstruction Pass on Orcas Island is so special that one of the former editors of this book became engaged there. He and his now-wife watched the sun set over the sound from a rock they were sitting on, and just before the sun disappeared behind the island, he proposed. After she said yes, seven otters swam by in succession, diving and catching fish and breaking clams open on their bellies. The otters then dove together and came up in a perfect semicircle around them. The otters, he says, looked them directly in the eye and barked before swimming out of sight. They took it as a sign.

This is a place of quiet beauty and simple pleasures. I should say up front that it is not exactly tent camping but more like baby backpacking, with less than a mile to walk to your campsite. Like Rialto Beach (see page 40), it's a perfect introduction for those new to backpacking—a light trek that is more than worth the burden of your pack. Both places also have water views. But that's where the similarity ends.

The morning view from the water's edge, down a flight of stairs from the campsites

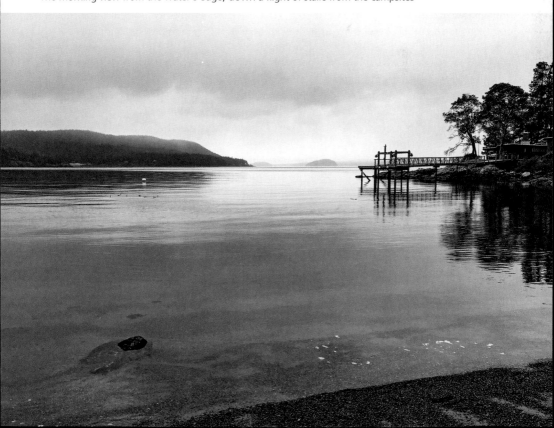

## KEY INFORMATION

**CONTACT:** 360-376-2326, Obstruction Pass State Park; 360-902-8844, Washington State Parks; parks.state.wa.us

**OPEN:** Year-round

**SITES:** 9 primitive, 1 marine trail

**EACH SITE HAS:** Picnic table, fire pit

**ASSIGNMENT:** First come, first served; no reservations

**REGISTRATION:** Self-registration at the bottom of the trail

**AMENITIES:** 2 vault toilets at the top of the trail and 2 at the trailhead, nonpotable water, no garbage facilities (campers must carry in and carry out)

**PARKING:** At trailhead, 0.5 mile from campground

**FEE:** $12 per site, plus $10 per vehicle to park at the trailhead

**ELEVATION:** Sea level

---

**RESTRICTIONS:**

**PETS:** On leash only

**FIRES:** In grated pits only

**VEHICLES:** Sites are approximately 0.5 mile from the parking lot

**ALCOHOL:** Permitted

From the trailhead, three footpaths descend through 80 acres of old-growth forest. The main and cliff-face trails make a lollipop loop with each other, while a third, newer trail sweeps east around the edge of the park. The main trail is 0.6 mile; the cliff-face trail, affording views of the water from a bluff on the way, is 0.4 mile and meets up with the main trail halfway down, for a total of 0.7 mile. The upper trail is slightly longer but still less than a mile. This pocket of rainforest on the east side of the island is lush and vibrant three seasons out of the year. In the summer it dries out a bit, but compensation is found in the thickets of foxglove and lupine reaching well over head height. In the summer, the dappled sunlight explodes on these patches of purple splashed across the forest floor in any opening wide enough to let light in. Cedar and Douglas-fir, hemlock, and spruce dominate the graywacke-studded growth and are punctuated by alder and yew. Closer to the water, the shore is thick with madrone, the red-barked icon of Northwest coasts. The main beach is a gem: a 150-yard crescent of soft pebbles and driftwood. The rocks are smooth and multicolored, and the beach offers views of the strait. The best experience is past the main beach, however, where a rock juts into the water with private pebbled beaches on either side. Eagles and ospreys abound, and the air is full of the screeching of Steller's jays. Seals are not uncommon. Purple-and-orange starfish cling to the rocks at low tide, and crabs in a hundred colors scuttle from shadow to shadow.

Some of the fairly secluded campsites at Obstruction Pass have views of the water. They're on the main trail just before it reaches the beach. Two are at the top of the trail and two are at the bottom. Because reservations are not accepted, campers are advised to arrive early on the day they wish to camp, keeping in mind that alternative accommodations on Orcas Island are likely to be quite expensive.

Obstruction Pass is beautiful all year. The islands get less rain and more sun than most of western Washington, but it's still the Northwest coast, and campers should be prepared for wet weather, brisk temperatures, and steady wind no matter when they visit. I recommend a weekday visit to Obstruction Pass. On the weekend, local high school students descend on the park, and it can be a bit noisy, but during the week it's a haven.

Obstruction Pass is part of the Cascadia Marine Trail. It's easily accessible by kayak and an excellent staging area for paddling exploration of the San Juans.

This is a unique and relatively unknown gem. It's home to an array of wildlife, and if you're lucky, you may see some of the more reclusive inhabitants: a pod of orcas, or the island's mythical herd of white deer.

## Obstruction Pass State Park Campground

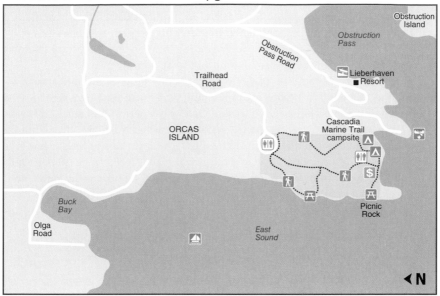

## GETTING THERE

Take the Washington State Ferry from Anacortes, WA, or Sidney, BC, to Orcas Island. Follow the signs to Eastsound, about 8 miles, and turn right onto Main Street, traveling through town as it becomes Crescent Beach Drive. After about 1 mile, turn right onto Olga Road. Follow the signs to Olga, about 6.5 miles. Turn left on Point Lawrence Road and then right on Obstruction Pass Road, then right again on Trailhead Road—a poorly marked gravel road. The park is at the end of the road, a little less than a mile. Total driving is 17–18 miles from the ferry landing.

**GPS COORDINATES** N48° 36.150'  W122° 49.500'

# 19

# ⛺ Shaw County Park Campground

Beauty ★★★★ Privacy ★★★★ Spaciousness ★★★★ Quiet ★★★★★ Security ★★★★★ Cleanliness ★★★★★

*Sunsets over Shaw Island are beautiful, and if you're lucky, you just might get to hear the orcas sing.*

Shaw County Park Campground on Shaw Island is another excellent base camp for paddling the San Juans. The smallest of the four islands with ferry service, Shaw has only 250 residents. There's a general store at the ferry landing, but beyond that, the island has no commercial ventures of any kind. Plan to camp and to do your own cooking.

The park is unique because of its sandy beach. Sandy beaches are uncommon in the Northwest, and this one is a beauty, with the finest sand you'll find anywhere. The beach curves in a long arc around Indian Cove, a calm, shallow bay perfect for launching kayaks.

The 12 campsites are tucked in the trees along the water. At night, the sound of the water lapping in and out is audible from all the sites. A waterfront site with a view is going to be ideal (sites 1–6); a wooded site across the gravel road is just as nice (sites 10 and 11), as you're still mere feet from the water. If you come on foot, by bike, or by kayak, you can pay for one of the Care to Share spots in site 9, which are reserved solely for guests traveling

South Beach campsites offer views of Puget Sound and Canoe and Lopez Islands beyond.

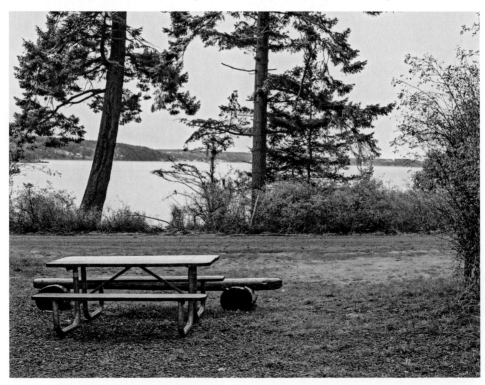

## KEY INFORMATION

**CONTACT:** 360-378-8420 or parks@ sanjuanco.com, San Juan County Parks; 360-468-4673, park manager; sanjuanco .com/523/Shaw-Island

**OPEN:** Year-round

**SITES:** 12; groups can call to reserve sites 10 and 11, which function as a group site that accommodates up to 15 people and up to 4 vehicles (included in the fee)

**EACH SITE HAS:** Fire pit

**ASSIGNMENT:** First come, first served. Reservations accepted and recommended during summer months for 10 of the 12 sites but not necessary

**REGISTRATION:** Self-registration on-site, online, and by phone

**AMENITIES:** 2 vault toilets, 3 water spigots (seasonal), water fountain, pavilion, boat launch, baseball/softball diamond

**PARKING:** At individual sites

**FEE:** $16–$21 standard (up to 4 people), $6–$9 each additional person, $3 each additional person aged 5–11, $5–$6 Care to Share site, $43 group site, $9–$11 each additional vehicle (price depends on season), $5 per person fee for failing to register

**ELEVATION:** Sea level

---

## RESTRICTIONS:

**PETS:** On leash only, owners must clean up after them

**QUIET HOURS:** 10 p.m.–7 a.m.

**FIRES:** In pits only, wood gathering prohibited

**VEHICLES:** Maximum 2 cars per site, no more than 4 people per car, private property at either end of the beach

**ALCOHOL:** Permitted

---

without a motorized vehicle. This makes the park an ideal place for kayakers to stop for the night, as they avoid the ferry charge and pay only a nominal fee for the site. The idea is that we share our resources, and people who care enough not to drive a car or powerboat receive consideration for chipping in. The park is a stop on the Cascadia Marine Trail; many of the campgrounds along this trail offer Care to Share sites.

The park has fair amenities for such a small campground. The pavilion is a common roofed area with tables, a woodstove, and a phone for emergency use with important numbers posted beside it. It's situated on a lawn that, while not flat enough for a game of Frisbee, is suitable for playing catch. Campers are prohibited from gathering firewood, but bundles are available for a nominal fee. If you want to avoid paying for it, bring your own wood with you.

Register at the self-registration booth on the left side of the road about halfway to the beach. Check-in begins at noon. Guests are advised to check the registration booth for availability before pitching their tents. Campers should be aware that the areas at either end of the beach are private property. People live on Shaw because they want privacy, and that should be respected.

Shaw is an excellent place for biking. The island is flat, and with few people, traffic is light even in the summer. Bikers and pedestrians can take advantage of 14 miles of public roads. There are dozens of quiet bays easily accessible on foot or by bike. If you're feeling sociable, consider visiting Our Lady of the Rock Monastery, home to a Benedictine order that focuses on service to the people of the islands and stewardship of the land. The order has a 300-acre property and raises crops, sheep, cattle, and llamas. As much as possible, the nuns are self-sufficient, raising their own food, including poultry, vegetables, and herbs. They also produce fine woolens from their sheep and alpacas. The property is stunning, and the nuns are warm and open.

At low tide, Indian Cove becomes a broad flat of tidepools ideal for children and beach-combers. For much of the year, the shallow water hosts dozens of blue herons, which stalk silently as the shadows lengthen toward sunset.

## Shaw County Park Campground

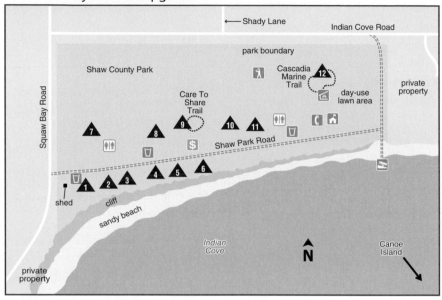

## GETTING THERE

Take the Washington State Ferry from Anacortes, WA, or Sidney, BC, to Shaw Island. From the ferry landing, follow Blind Bay Road south 1.5 miles, and turn left on Squaw Bay Road. After 0.5 mile, turn left onto a gravel road marked CAMPING. Officially, this is Shaw Park Road, but it's unmarked. Sites are on both sides of the road.

**GPS COORDINATES** N48° 33.940' W122° 56.232'

# 20

# Spencer Spit State Park Campground

Beauty ★★★★★ Privacy ★★★★ Spaciousness ★★★★ Quiet ★★★★★ Security ★★★ Cleanliness ★★★★

*If you want to see the beautiful San Juan Islands archipelago, this is the place to stay. You can camp right on the beach.*

A book about car camping in the Northwest would not be complete without fully representing the San Juan Archipelago's several options. Including Lopez Island is relatively easy, actually, despite the fact that the San Juans unofficially include 768 exposed rocks, reefs, and islands.

For starters, only 175 of these land formations have been named, and 85 are inaccessible to the public, protected by their designation as the San Juan Islands National Wildlife Refuge. Only five can be reached by ferry either from Anacortes, Washington, on the US side or Sidney, British Columbia, on the Canadian side. Of these, only four maintained campgrounds are accessible by car, one of which is Spencer Spit State Park on Lopez Island. There are many boat-in only campgrounds throughout the islands, including Griffon Bay State Park and Posey Island State Park, which you should further research for a quieter, more rustic, and more strenuous way to experience the islands.

Far from the seasonal rat race and the citylike atmosphere of the much larger but filled-to-overflowing facilities on Orcas and San Juan islands, Spencer Spit is an excellent base camp for enjoying Lopez and its sister islands by car, foot, or bicycle. The only drawback to lovely little Spencer Spit is the same drawback that plagues all the other islands served by the same mode of transit: the Washington State Ferries.

What Spencer Spit's walk-in beach campsites lack in privacy they make up for in surroundings—you can see Flower, Blakely, and Orcas Islands in one direction and the spit in the other.

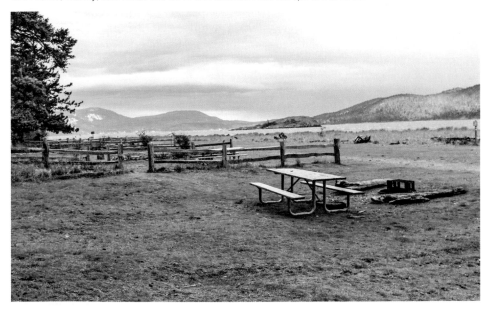

## KEY INFORMATION

**CONTACT:** 360-468-2251, Spencer Spit State Park; 360-902-8844, Washington State Parks; parks.state.wa.us

**OPEN:** March 2–October 29

**SITES:** 37 standard, 7 hiker/biker, 2 group camps (up to 20 people, up to 50 people), 7 walk-in beach sites

**EACH SITE HAS:** Picnic table, fire pit with grill

**ASSIGNMENT:** First come, first served; reservations accepted March 2–October 29, at 888-CAMPOUT (888-226-7688)

**REGISTRATION:** Self-registration on-site, online, by phone

**AMENITIES:** Bathhouse with sinks and toilets (no showers); dump station

**PARKING:** In campground and at some individual sites, parking for beach sites near trailhead

**FEE:** $30–$35 standard, $12 primitive

**ELEVATION:** Sea level

---

**RESTRICTIONS:**

**PETS:** On leash only

**FIRES:** In fire pits only

**ALCOHOL:** Permitted

**VEHICLES:** Self-contained RVs up to 28', no hookups

First, plan on becoming a veritable scholar of the ferry schedule. Pick one up when you pay at the tollbooth. Make sure you know that where you want to go is also where the ferry is planning to go. Ditto on when. In the summertime, additional ferries are put on high-volume routes to accommodate the heavy onslaught of tourists and vacationers. This does not mean that all ferries stop at all islands all the time, however. Some ferries stop at some of the islands some of the time. Lopez is one of those "some of the time" islands.

One of the most appealing aspects of Spencer Spit State Park is that you can camp right on the beach—in designated areas, of course. You'll have to pack your gear down from the parking lot above. With the park's reputation for excellent crabbing and clamming, it's worth considering making some of that gear the items you'll need to catch your dinner—a bucket or two, a sand shovel, a crab net, bait, a cooking pot. Maybe it seems a bit cumbersome, but the rewards make the effort a distant memory. Plus, the campground provides wheelbarrows to help you lug your stuff to the lower beachfront campsites.

Lopez Island is, in my estimation, the premier bicycling island of the San Juans and can easily be covered in a day of riding if you're accustomed to 40 miles or so. Except for the hill up from the ferry terminal, which you'll most likely ascend by car anyway, Lopez features mildly rolling farmland with paved roads and a noticeable lack of traffic—even on weekends. It's possible that you'll encounter more bicycles than cars on any given day during the summer.

One of my favorite pastimes on Lopez is riding out to Shark Reef Park with the three Bs—a book, binoculars, and a brown-bag lunch—to watch the sea lions that sprawl en masse on the offshore rocks. From your vantage point at Shark Reef, you can also look far across the San Juan Channel to windswept Cattle Point on San Juan Island, where the only sand dunes in the entire island group exist.

Other points of interest on Lopez Island include the village of Lopez, which has some excellent restaurants, interesting shops, and a small museum. Richardson and Mackaye Harbor at the island's southern tip are also highly scenic spots easily reached by car or bicycle. The ferry from Lopez takes you directly into Friday Harbor on San Juan Island and Orcas on (what else?) Orcas Island, both thriving business districts. Unless you're interested in touring the other islands extensively, it's faster and cheaper just to walk onto the ferry from Lopez and kick around Friday Harbor and Orcas on foot.

The climate of the San Juan Islands is unique. Although westerly marine winds can bring a change in the weather at any time, the islands fall under the Olympic Mountains' rain shadow, which extends northeast across the Strait of Juan de Fuca. As a result, rainfall averages only about 15 to 25 inches per year. Summers can be quite hot—some of my deepest tans are from San Juan bicycle trips—and the lovely, balmy days of autumn are unsurpassed. Even in summer, however, nights are chilly enough for a campfire to be appreciated.

## Spencer Spit State Park Campground

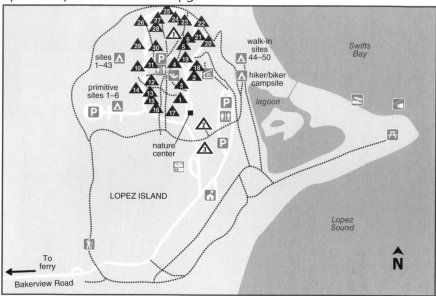

## GETTING THERE

Take a ferry from the Anacortes terminal to Lopez Island. The ride to Lopez is less than 45 minutes one way. From the ferry terminal at the northern end of Lopez Island, take Ferry Road south, and follow the signs to the park. The total distance from the ferry terminal is barely 5 miles.

**GPS COORDINATES** N48° 32.200' W122° 51.598'

# NORTHERN CASCADES AND ENVIRONS

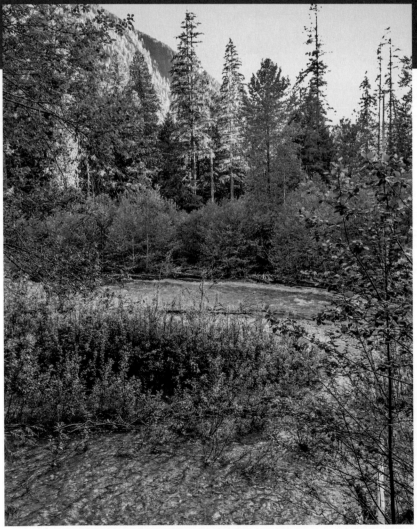

North Fork Cascade River, Mineral Park Campground (see page 91)

# 21

# ⚠ Buck Creek Campground

Beauty ★★★★ Privacy ★★★★ Spaciousness ★★★ Quiet ★★★★★ Security ★★★★ Cleanliness ★★★★★

*The creek is the centerpiece of this nearly lost campground, where staying put is as tempting as hiking.*

Some campgrounds are great base camps because of their proximity to a trailhead or other premium destination. They may be bare bones, but they get you where you want to be. Other base camps invite you to stay put—you almost forget why you came out here in the first place. If I wanted the bulk of my camping trip to be about relaxing in my campsite, dipping my toes in the water, and reading in my hammock, I would choose Buck Creek.

Buck Creek Campground was almost lost entirely in the floods of 2003 and 2006. After a decade-long closure, it has finally reopened along with the roads that lead to it. The campground still has room for improvement (nearly half of it remains closed), but I couldn't let it go unmentioned. It's a stunning place to unfurl a sleeping bag in this newly reaccessible section of Mount Baker–Snoqualmie National Forest.

Just because I would be content to lounge around my campsite, that isn't to say there's nothing else to do. (See nearby Sulphur Creek Campground, page 100, for more information.) This is a marvelous outpost for other adventures: birding, fishing, uncrowded hiking, and general meandering.

Buck Creek, near campsite 4

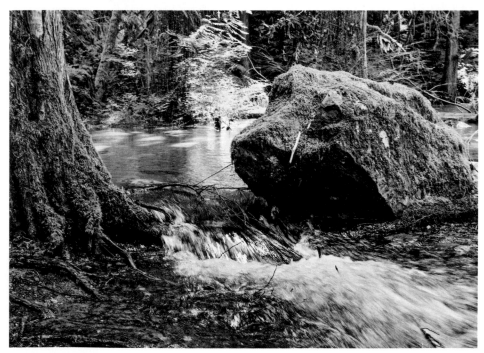

## KEY INFORMATION

**CONTACT:** 360-436-1155, Darrington Ranger Station, tinyurl.com/buckcreekcampground

**OPEN:** Year-round

**SITES:** 15 (1 is a double site for up to 12 people)

**EACH SITE HAS:** Picnic table, fire pit with grill

**ASSIGNMENT:** First come, first served; reservations accepted for some sites

**REGISTRATION:** Self-registration on-site, online, and by phone

**AMENITIES:** Vault toilets, nonpotable water

**PARKING:** At individual sites

**FEE:** $14 single, $7 each additional vehicle, $25 double site, $5 day use

**ELEVATION:** 1,361'

---

**RESTRICTIONS:**

**PETS:** On leash only

**FIRES:** In fire pits only

**ALCOHOL:** Permitted

**VEHICLES:** Large RVs and trailers not recommended

Hike Buck Creek trail right from the campground for better views of the creek, or check out Huckleberry Mountain (back down Siuattle Road from where you came) if you're into hiking straight up for good views. There's also Canyon Lake, Green Mountain, and Milk Creek, a 34-mile trail that leads you along the PCT for part of the way. Backcountry stays require a permit, which you can get at the Darrington Ranger Station. Each of these trails has had varying degrees of maintenance because of washouts, landslides, and flooding and are being repaired over time. Check trail conditions before you go and avoid fording rivers if they're too unruly. Consider hiking with poles for the added stability.

Buck Creek is a powerful force coursing through the campground. The creek was wide and fast when I visited in the late spring of 2017. All of the campsites were dappled in sunshine and most of them border the creek. About half of the loop was closed when I was there, and it was unclear how soon it would be reopened. That aside, the campground is beautiful and primitive. There isn't much here in the way of amenities (vault toilets and no drinking water), so some might pass it by. Site 7 is by far my favorite. From here, looking up and down the creek, all feels right in the world.

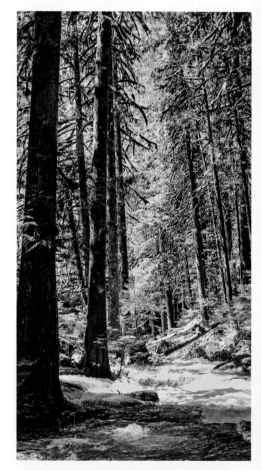

Buck Creek runs along the southern edge of the campground, which has no shortage of trees.

This spot is secluded and quiet (aside from the sound of rushing water). Even with some sites off-limits, it fulfills my core requirements for a perfect tent-camping experience. Camp hosts are usually stationed here Memorial Day–Labor Day. They're bound to be a good resource for which trails are in good shape when you visit.

I'm so grateful to all the people who spent years working to reopen the road, the campground, and the trails in this area. These dedicated folks—when the road was closed—biked, hiked, hauled packs of tools, and volunteered hundreds of hours in order to preserve Green Mountain Lookout. Although on the National Register of Historic Places, the lookout was at risk. This is just one example. Every time I'm out on a trail, especially one a little worse for wear, I think of all the people who have helped create and maintain our amazing hiking opportunities in the Northwest. Washington has so many trails and Forest Service roads to maintain—this section of the forest could have easily been closed off indefinitely. Luckily, it's open and it's summoning us.

## Buck Creek Campground

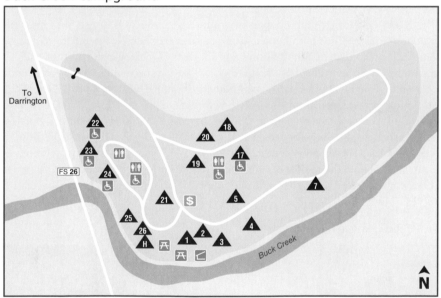

## GETTING THERE

From Darrington, head north on WA 530 about 7 miles. Turn right onto NF 26/Suiattle River Road. The campground will be on the left after 15 miles. Be aware that the road is gravel for the last stretch.

**GPS COORDINATES** N48° 16.100' W121° 19.700'

# 22

# ⛺ Colonial Creek Campground

Beauty ★★★★ Privacy ★★★ Spaciousness ★★★★ Quiet ★★★ Security ★★★★★ Cleanliness ★★★★★

*Enjoy views of glaciated peaks above turquoise water, and hike to your heart's content.*

If it's beauty you're after, I can't suggest a better place. The water is a mesmerizing turquoise and the mountain views are breathtaking. I'd venture to guess that most people driving the scenic North Cascades Highway (WA 20) feel compelled to pull over the moment they catch their first glimpse of Diablo Lake. So why not camp here?

While Colonial Creek is a bigger and busier campground than I'd normally insist you try, it strikes a balance between simple to get to and scenic as all get-out. It's worth rubbing elbows with your neighbors, and that's a lot coming from me. Don't worry, the campsites are well spaced and spacious, depending on which one you nab. Even though a reservation system applies to the South Loop's 100 sites during the main season, the North Loop's 42 sites are always first come, first served.

The North Loop and South Loop campgrounds straddle WA 20 and both have campsites along the water. The South Loop's waterside sites are snug—we're talking sardine snug in some cases. Though I'm almost always a proponent of picking a site on the water, I recommend the forest here. You'll be drawn to visit the water no matter where you're cooking and camping. For the South Loop, I recommend the upper walk-in sites (129–141). They feel the most private, and from this patch of forest, you almost forget you're in a larger campground. You have to walk your gear in on the trail (50–100 yards), but it's worth it for the small sanctuary that privacy provides. If you'd prefer not to haul gear (or if those spots are taken), consider a site on a "corner," like 137 or 142. I stayed in one and couldn't see or hear my neighbors in the middle of summer. If you've come for the water and you must be on the water, the waterfront walk-in sites on the North Loop are a bit better spaced.

View of Diablo Lake from Thunder Creek Trail

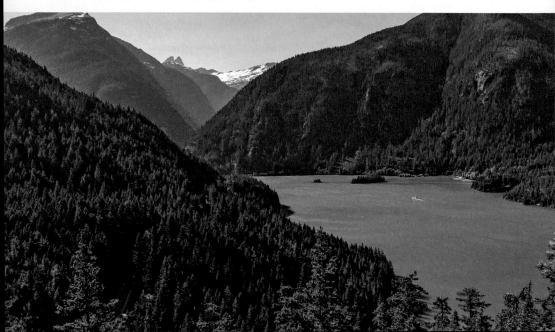

## KEY INFORMATION

**CONTACT:** 360-854-7200, North Cascades National Park; recreation.gov

**OPEN:** Year-round, limited sites and services available during winter months

**SITES:** 142

**EACH SITE HAS:** Picnic table, fire pit with grill

**ASSIGNMENT:** First come, first served; reservations accepted for South Loop campground at recreation.gov and 877-444-6777

**REGISTRATION:** On-site, online, and by phone

**AMENITIES:** Flush toilets (vault toilets in winter), potable water, dump station, garbage and recycling service, walk-in sites, fishing pier, boat launch, animal-proof storage lockers near walk-in sites

**PARKING:** At individual sites and near access to walk-in sites

**FEE:** $16

**ELEVATION:** 1,233'

---

**RESTRICTIONS:**

**PETS:** On leash only

**FIRES:** In fire pits only, wood gathering prohibited

**ALCOHOL:** Permitted

**VEHICLES:** Small trailers only (limited side clearance)

As soon as you pitch your tent, you're going to want to go down to the lake. It lures me in every time I see it. I could sit myself in a chair all day, just staring at the sun glinting on the surface and the glaciers in the distance. North Cascades National Park has more than 300 glaciers—that's hundreds more than Glacier National Park—making it the most glaciated of any US park outside Alaska. Several glaciers feed into Diablo Lake, including Boston Glacier, the park's largest. Glaciers here are not immune to a loss of volume due to climate change. Researchers and monitoring programs have been collecting data for decades. It's worth looking up aerial photographs of the area to see how much it's changed over the years. The beautiful, bold turquoise color of the lake is thanks to the surrounding glaciers, which supply the water with glacial flour—finely ground particles of rock. These particles reflect light so the water appears a stunning aquamarine, teal, turquoise, or green depending on the day, the angle of the sun, the size of the particles, how many are suspended, and where you're standing when you look at the lake.

The water is cold, but you can swim right from the beach in the campground (or launch a human-powered boat or small motorized boat). You might also enjoy the water from a height as you hike along Thunder Knob Trail for a shorter hike (3.6 miles) with a big view, or Thunder Creek Trail for a more extended exploration with lots of opportunities to view the lake and the surrounding snowcapped mountains of the Cascades. The trail (12 miles round-trip) is flat for much of the way but eventually climbs a steep slope, and the water looks especially nice from up above. You can see Diablo Dam from the ridge as you're hiking.

Whatever outings you have planned in this region of the North Cascades, Colonial Creek is a great place to take respite. There are interpretive trails as well as a ranger station. Rangers are always extremely helpful in pointing out a great hike and giving you bonus factoids about the region. Newhalem is the closest town where you can get supplies (and there's a visitor center there). You may even want to take the ferry up to Ross Lake Resort, where you can rent a kayak and paddle around. I should mention that a number of great spots along Diablo Lake and Ross Lake have boat-in campgrounds (often with as few as three sites). If that's more your thing, stop at the information center in Marblemount for the required backcountry permit. Opportunities for quaint, private, rustic camping abound.

## GETTING THERE

From I-5, drive 65 miles east on WA 20. Turn right into the campground, just beyond mile marker 130.

**GPS COORDINATES** N48° 41.350'  W121° 05.733'

## Colonial Creek North Loop Campground

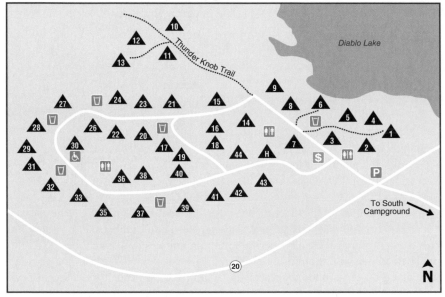

## Colonial Creek South Loop Campground

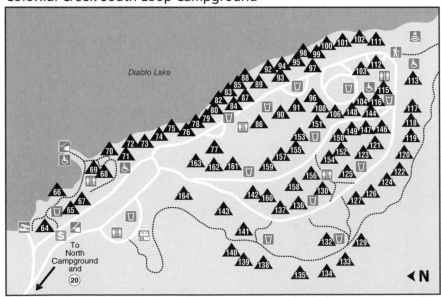

# 23

# ⚡ Falls Creek Campground

Beauty ★★★★ Privacy ★★★ Spaciousness ★★★★★ Quiet ★★★★★ Security ★★★ Cleanliness ★★★★★

*Falls Creek is not far from the bustle of western-style Winthrop but is on a good fishing stream and has a roaring waterfall nearby.*

Don't try to figure it out. Chewuch. I mean Chewack. No, Chewuck. Or is it Chewuk? Chewak? OK, enough. I don't really know which is correct and apparently neither does anyone else in the state. You'll find all varieties on maps and road signs and in reference books and guidebooks. Some maps even use Chewuch and Chewack side by side. There is consistency in the inconsistency, at least.

Perhaps the confusion dates back to as early as the mid-1800s when the Chewuch River (I'm making an executive decision here) first appeared as such on maps of the region. This area of the Methow Valley was just starting to open up to mining activity at about that time, but it's likely the explorers and traders who preceded this frenzy were responsible for naming the natural features as they went. As with many parts of Washington, history was not recorded until there was an actual settlement in any given place; so much of what we know about earlier times is gleaned from the journals and diaries of adventurous souls who came seeking their fortunes—or at least an interesting route to them.

The Chewuch River Valley has remained relatively undeveloped since its first discovery because it's overshadowed by the more prominent, much-publicized Methow Valley with

The Chewuch River as it passes through Falls Creek Campground in autumn

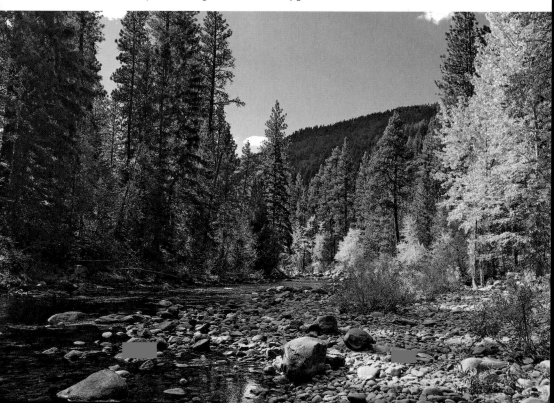

## KEY INFORMATION

**CONTACT:** 509-664-9200, Okanogan-Wenatchee National Forest; 509-996-4000, Methow Valley Visitor Center; tinyurl.com/fallscreekcampground

**OPEN:** May–October

**SITES:** 7

**EACH SITE HAS:** Picnic table, fire pit with grill

**ASSIGNMENT:** First come, first served

**REGISTRATION:** On-site

**AMENITIES:** Vault toilets (ADA-compliant), garbage service, potable water in summer, accessible trail to falls across road, no trash receptacles

**PARKING:** At individual sites

**FEE:** $8, $5 each additional vehicle

**ELEVATION:** 2,100'

---

**RESTRICTIONS:**

**PETS:** On leash only

**FIRES:** In fire pits only

**ALCOHOL:** Permitted

**VEHICLES:** Trailers and RVs up to 18'

western-style Winthrop at its epicenter. Gracing the land throughout is the meandering charm of the crystal-clear Methow River as it makes its way southeast to the Columbia River through rolling rangelands dotted with groves of cottonwood, aspen, tamarack, and pine. These days, explorers to the Methow (pronounced "MET-how") Valley come in the form of well-fleeced outdoor enthusiasts lured from the wet side of the mountains in their Range Rovers and Subarus to the dry, sun-drenched eastern brink of the North Cascades.

Finding the Chewuch River and, ultimately, Falls Creek Campground, is as easy as looking down at it when you drive over the bridge that brings you into Winthrop from the west on WA 20. Turn left at the intersection, try not to pick off a pedestrian from the throngs, battle your way to the end of town, and continue north. Either the Eastside Chewuch Road or the West Chewuch Road take you where you need to go; just follow the signs to FS 51. In no time, you'll feel the claustrophobic impact of "TMT" (too many tourists) slip away as you beat feet up the narrow Chewuch River canyon to your destination.

I must warn you: the upper Chewuch Valley has been "charred up" by forest fires, and the scene farther up FS 51 and FS 5160 to road's end at Thirtymile Campground (what's left of it) is a shocker. This was the site of the tragic Thirtymile Fire, which took the lives of U.S. Forest Service workers in July 2001, and was also part of a second blaze—the Farewell Fire—which destroyed 81,000 acres in August 2003. A memorial honors the four who gave their lives trying to combat the Thirtymile blaze, which was started by—it grieves me to say—an uncontrolled cooking fire. Farewell was started by lightning and roared out of control for nearly six weeks, costing $36 million and making it the largest Pacific Northwest fire in the disastrously dry 2003 season. The giant fires of the 2016 and 2017 seasons will have lasting impacts on Washington as well.

Fortunately, Falls Creek Campground was just outside the fire line and is the embodiment of the campgrounds that fell victim inside the line. Simple, rustic, and unadorned with human amenities—except for a hand pump and vault toilet—it's richly quiet with the sounds of the Chewuch shushing by, the warm summer wind sighing in the pines, birds twittering, and chipmunks chiding. Beds of pine needles make for soft tent pads. Large sites with parking spaces away from the camp area afford privacy, and low-growing shrubbery present a clean, uncluttered profile.

With only seven sites from which to choose (all stretched along the curving bank of the Chewuch), it's splitting hairs to say which one is best. If sites 3, 4, or 5 are available, this puts you closest to the river and away from either end of the camp road where it leaves and returns to FS 51. Each of the sites feels private if a little open (not much vegetation to speak of here), and the river babbles loudly in each of them.

Staying at Falls Creek Campground gives you the daily treat of Falls Creek Falls, across the road and up an accessible 0.25-mile trail—nature's open-air shower. After a hot, dusty mountain scramble on foot or by bike, the tumult of water falling off the end of Eightmile Ridge sends delicious spray cascading over you as you approach the grotto.

The Forest Service is restoring many of the trails and trailheads that were consumed by fire and were once popular jump-offs into Pasayten Wilderness in the upper Chewuch. It's worth checking the USFS website for which terrain is in the best condition this season. Check out Falls Creek Falls (a 4-mile round-trip hike) or North Twentymile Peak nearby. There are also hiking options up FS 37 in the Tiffany Mountain area above the Boulder Creek and North Fork Salmon Creek watersheds. Though not as large a roadless area as the hallowed Pasayten, Tiffany Mountain has been considered for Research Natural Area status because it has unique ecosystems.

In the tradition of a bygone era, explore away!

## Falls Creek Campground

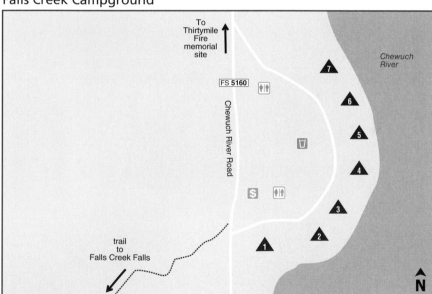

## GETTING THERE

From Winthrop, drive 6.5 miles north on CR 1213 (West Chewuch Road). Then continue north 5 miles on FS 51 and FS 5160 to the campground.

**GPS COORDINATES** N48° 38.241' W120° 09.308'

# 24

# Hart's Pass Campground

Beauty ★★★★★ Privacy ★★★ Spaciousness ★★★ Quiet ★★★★★ Security ★★★ Cleanliness ★★★★

*Remote and spectacularly beautiful, this small tent-only campground is an outdoor adventurer's dream. Get there before the snow!*

Mention the name Hart's Pass to just about anyone who considers himself or herself a well-traveled outdoor adventurer in the Northwest, and watch their eyes glaze over.

When I first started asking around for campground suggestions in the North Cascades years ago, I got as many different suggestions as the number of people I asked. Except they would always end by saying, almost as an afterthought, so they wouldn't risk offending me, and with a cautious sidelong glance, "Of course, you've already got Hart's Pass?" Something between a question and a statement.

For those of you who thought you were somehow going to be able to keep this magical place to yourself, I'm sorry. Hart's Pass continues to delight and amaze those discovering it for the first time and the rest of us who won't let go. While the campground is tiny and can accommodate only five independent parties, there are plenty of open spaces in the mix of peaks and meadows and forests and trails in just about every direction to lose yourself and get away from the pack. In no time, you'll be rambling the heady altitudes of this prototypical North Cascades terrain in isolated bliss.

View near Hart's Pass, not far from Slate Peak Lookout

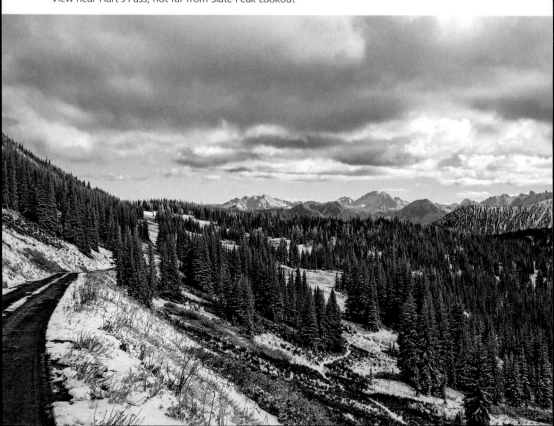

## KEY INFORMATION

**CONTACT:** 509-664-9200, Okanogan-Wenatchee National Forest; 509-996-4000, Methow Valley Visitor Center; tinyurl.com/hartspasscampground

**OPEN:** Mid-July–late September

**SITES:** 5

**EACH SITE HAS:** Picnic table, fire ring

**ASSIGNMENT:** First come, first served; no reservations

**REGISTRATION:** Self-registration on-site

**AMENITIES:** Vault toilets (wheelchair accessible), no water

**PARKING:** In campground

**FEE:** $8, $5 each additional vehicle

**ELEVATION:** 6,210'

**RESTRICTIONS:**

**PETS:** On leash only

**FIRES:** In fire pits only

**ALCOHOL:** Permitted

**VEHICLES:** Trailers and RVs not permitted (roads do not allow)

**OTHER:** Pack out garbage

---

What Hart's Pass Campground has going for it in a big way is this is the veritable western edge of the massive Pasayten Wilderness, a 505,524-acre roadless tract extending north to the US-Canada border and east to the ridgetops above the Okanogan Valley. Within this territory are 1,000 miles of trails, many of them unmaintained and leading into some of the most difficult terrain in the entire Washington Cascades. Out of the metamorphic rock, Ice Age glaciers produced an intimidating collection of razorlike ridges, deep valley troughs, cirques, and couloirs that test the most skilled mountaineers.

If you're not quite up to tackling nature at its rugged best, try a simpler approach with a drive up to Slate Peak Lookout. This is the highest point in Washington that is accessible by car. Once one of 93 manned U.S. Forest Service lookouts in the North Cascades, Slate Peak (7,488') offers identification displays of the peaks, passes, and ridges visible from its 360-degree viewing area.

Passing near camp, the Pacific Crest Trail is the major north–south thoroughfare for foot travel. Follow it in either direction for further samples of North Cascades beauty. Wide meadows burst with nearly six dozen flowering varieties of plant life at the height of their bloom (at this altitude and latitude, that tends to be late July to mid-August).

The road into Hart's Pass from Mazama (a tedious 12 miles) is not recommended for extra-wide or low-clearance vehicles. For those of you daring enough to continue beyond Hart's Pass by car, some points of historical interest will reward your perseverance. I'll warn you now that the road gets even rougher down into the Slate Creek Valley, where evidence of mining activity from the 1880s and 1890s still lingers. Down the road from Chancellor, en route to Barron, is an abandoned building that once served as the stage stop and post office for the mining community before the Hart's Pass Road was built. If you can get there, the area around Chancellor and Barron is worth investigation.

A word of caution about traveling to these remote North Cascades destinations: Mazama offers little in the way of services, and there is really nothing substantial between Winthrop to the east on WA 20 and Marblemount to the west—a stretch of 100 spectacularly scenic but civilization-free miles.

Despite its ranking as one of the 10 most scenic drives in the United States, North Cascades Highway is not open year-round. It's usually the first of the east–west highways to close due to heavy snowfall, and it's normally off-limits November–April. You may want to beat the snow with an early fall camping trip to Hart's Pass just to take in the lovely autumn colors that adorn the length of the highway. I caught the fall colors in mid-September last year, but when I got to the campground, the scenery had shifted to a wintery mix. If you're thinking of going right after the snowmelt, keep in mind that the mosquitoes and horseflies will be at their worst then.

Travel tip: Hart's Pass is one of very few camping options in the area, and with only five sites—all first come, first served—you may find yourself having to take a number. Meadows Campground, about a mile due south of Hart's Pass on FS 500, has 14 sites. If both Hart's Pass and Meadows are full, the closest campgrounds are Ballard and River Bend back down on the Methow River.

If you decide you need to head back down that treacherous winding road, don't do so until you take in the view from Slate Peak. It's a stunner! And that's an understatement.

## Hart's Pass Campground

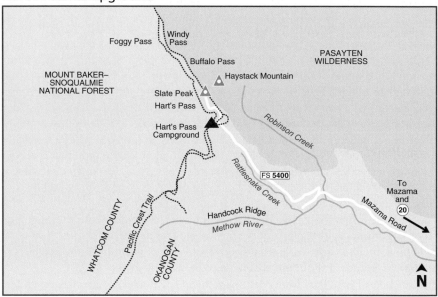

## GETTING THERE

From Mazama (about 15 miles northwest of Winthrop just off WA 20), follow Mazama Road (Lost Creek Road) about 6 miles to FS 5400. The campground is 12 slow, rough miles up FS 5400.

**GPS COORDINATES** N48° 43.250' W120° 40.200'

# 25

# ⛺ Mineral Park Campground

Beauty ★★★★ Privacy ★★★★ Spaciousness ★★★★ Quiet ★★★★ Security ★★★ Cleanliness ★★★★★

*This "secret" backdoor access that everyone knows about is a great base camp for exploring the wonders of North Cascades National Park.*

More than 30 years after I took my first drive over the North Cascades Highway and blistered myself from nose to toes going up the Sourdough Mountain Trail, I am discovering and rediscovering parts of the North Cascades that make me yearn for the sturdy legs, strong back, and gutsy determination that propelled me around these parts back then.

I think it took me this long to make my way to Mineral Park because in the height of my backcountry-tripping days, the phrases "Cascade Pass" and "absurdly crowded" were almost always mentioned in the same sentence. I never had any interest in Cascade River Road because it provided the easiest access to the most popular trail in the entire North Cascades National Park and associated recreation areas—the last place I wanted to be. I know some of you are shaking your heads in disbelief at this admission and what I've been missing. I know because I'm doing it too.

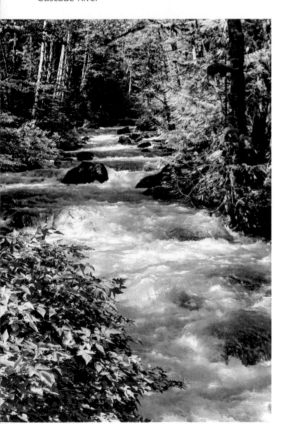

Cascade River

At any rate, I have finally ventured up Cascade River Road, twice now in the past year, and let me tell you, thank heaven for places like Mineral Park! Being a born-again car camper, I'm content to know that I'll be just getting back from my invigorating day hike to Cascade Pass and Sahale Arm (weekday only, as this remains an absurdly crowded weekend outing) and settling in for a quiet evening beside the swift-flowing Cascade River while the backpacking crowd fights over the few overloved high-country spots.

Located just outside the western boundary of North Cascades National Park South Unit, Mineral Park came as close as any campground can to being wiped out in the fall floods of 2003. This stretch of the Cascade River was particularly hard hit, and the devastation may be still evident, though much work has been done to repair the damage on land, including erecting steely new bridges to replace those that were probably pulverized into toothpicks and spit out downriver.

Mineral Park is actually two campgrounds split by the North Fork of the

## KEY INFORMATION

**CONTACT:** 541-338-7869, Hoodoo Recreation Services; 425-783-6000, Mount Baker–Snoqualmie National Forest; hoodoorecreation.com

**OPEN:** Memorial Day weekend–Labor Day weekend

**SITES:** 22 (8 east, 14 west)

**EACH SITE HAS:** Picnic table, fire pit with grill

**ASSIGNMENT:** First come, first served, or by reservation at 877-444-6777 or recreation.gov

**REGISTRATION:** On-site, online, or by phone

**AMENITIES:** Vault toilets, no potable water, garbage service

**PARKING:** At individual sites

**FEE:** $12 single, $20 double, $6 each additional vehicle

**ELEVATION:** 1,732'

**RESTRICTIONS:**

**PETS:** On leash only

**FIRES:** In fire pits only

**ALCOHOL:** Permitted

**VEHICLES:** Large RVs not recommended, small trailers OK

Cascade River as it merges with the South Fork to create the main Cascade River right in front of your eyes. The western area has more sites that are closer to the river, are more generously spaced, and have more of an open feel. The eastern area is a mix of individual and multiple sites lying beneath a canopy of evergreens, with a picnic area, several sites with a common parking area, and a lone site (8) in a pleasant little private glade on the shoulder of the North Fork.

Surprisingly, for a campground with few amenities, it's possible to reserve certain sites through the National Recreation Reservation System (see Key Information, above). Perhaps because Mineral Park is a national park access point, the Forest Service decided to offer reservations for a number of sites.

The terrain here is steep, and vertical hikes are the primary activity. Aside from the Cascade Pass Trail (which links with other routes within the North Cascades National Park network), there are less strenuous and involved choices for day hikes outside the park's domain, namely at Hidden Lakes and Monogram Lake (both of which are accessed via the Cascade River Road heading toward Marblemount). Chances are that there will be fewer people on these trails on any day of the week.

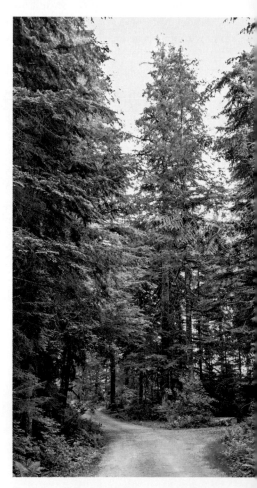

Evergreens tower above the campground road.

Fishing was probably decent at Mineral Park in the preflood era, but with the flow of the river altered dramatically by countless snags, fishing would be better attempted closer to the Skagit where it widens and the water-debris ratio favors the water.

For all intents and purposes, Mineral Park is a tent-camping delight even if you do nothing but sit by the river with a good book in hand. For armchair alpinists such as myself, I heartily recommend *North Cascades Crest: Notes and Images from America's Alps* by James Martin. Much of his discourse and photography record and reflect the glaciated heights just above and behind you.

## Mineral Park Campground

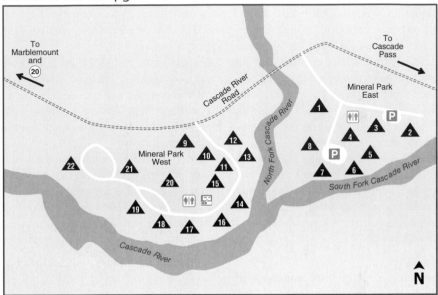

## GETTING THERE

From Marblemount, pick up Cascade River Road at the intersection where WA 20 takes a 90-degree bend to the east and the Cascade Road immediately crosses the Skagit River. Drive 15 miles on paved, then gravel, roads to the campground.

**GPS COORDINATES** N48° 27.816' W121° 10.022'

# 26

# Panorama Point Campground

Beauty ★★★★★ Privacy ★★★★ Spaciousness ★★★★ Quiet ★★★ Security ★★★★ Cleanliness ★★★★★

*This is a fisher's lake, but there's lots for others to do too.*

Many purist Northwest wilderness-goers purposefully overlook camping options at places like Baker Lake simply because they don't feel they will get a truly pristine experience if they can hear machines.

In the case of Panorama Point Campground midway up the western shore, that sound will most likely be the gentle buzz of small outboard motors as fishers put-put around in search of the best spots to hook their daily catch. They have their choice of such delights as rainbow, cutthroat, or Dolly Varden trout; kokanee salmon; and whitefish.

This is, indeed, a fisher's lake. But with miles and miles of U.S. Forest Service roads and trails to take you to soothing hot springs and deep into two designated wildernesses, a national recreation area, a national park, and an undeveloped eastern lakeshore, one can hardly complain that there's no getting away from things here. Just make sure you have a good Forest Service map and trail guides of the area before you find yourself at the mercy of the purists.

To the west of Panorama Point lies the glacier-encrusted mass of Mount Baker. This is Washington's third-highest volcano and is active only thermally as far as geologists can determine. Designated wilderness surrounds Mount Baker and is adjacent to national recreation areas on both north and south flanks of the mountain. Here you'll find unlimited hiking, backpacking, skiing, and climbing opportunities, depending on which season you choose to travel.

Kokanee salmon, whitefish, and several kinds of trout are found in Baker Lake.

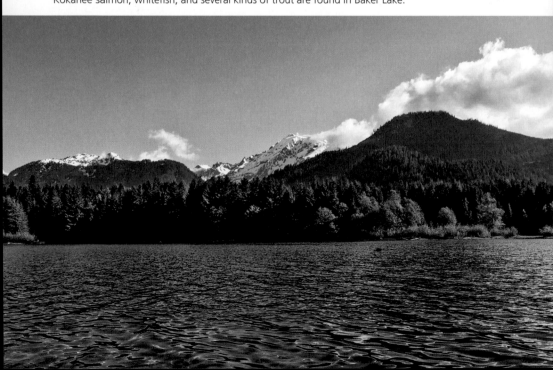

## KEY INFORMATION

**CONTACT:** 541-338-7869, Hoodoo Recreation Services; 425-783-6000, Mount Baker–Snoqualmie National Forest; hoodoorecreationservices.com

**OPEN:** May–mid-September

**SITES:** 15

**EACH SITE HAS:** Picnic table, fire pit with grill

**ASSIGNMENT:** First come, first served, or by reservation at 877-444-6777 or recreation.gov; reservations require a 3-day minimum stay

**REGISTRATION:** Self-registration on-site, online, or by phone

**AMENITIES:** Vault toilets; potable water; firewood; store, café, and ice within 1 mile; boat ramp nearby; no hookups

**PARKING:** At individual sites

**FEE:** $16 single, $30 double, $8 each additional vehicle

**ELEVATION:** 800'

**RESTRICTIONS:**

**PETS:** On leash only

**FIRES:** In fire pits only. Obtain firewood near the campground to prevent the spread of invasive species from outside sources.

**ALCOHOL:** Permitted

**VEHICLES:** Trailers and RVs up to 21'

**OTHER:** Permits required for overnight backpacking; parking permit required to park at trailhead

Check with the agencies that oversee these areas to find our if there are any special conditions and restrictions. Backpackers, for instance, will need permits for overnight trips into the backcountry.

North of the campground is the equally spectacular Mount Shuksan, a craggy sentinel of snow, ice, and rock that is the gateway for foot travelers approaching North Cascades National Park from the west. There could be no more fitting prototype to the challenging terrain than that embodied in names like Mount Despair, Damnation Park, Mount Challenger, Mount Terror, Mount Fury, and Jagged Ridge. These are but a few of the numerous natural shrines in the northern sector of North Cascades National Park that have been immortalized in the minds and journals of many a mountaineer.

East across Baker Lake is the smallest of the eight wilderness areas in the Mount Baker–Snoqualmie National Forest. Despite its diminutive size (14,300 acres), Noisy-Diobsud Wilderness is a place to be reckoned with. Elevations range from 2,000 to 6,234 feet, with only 2 miles of maintained trails. It's, for all intents and purposes, a place for experienced climbers and scramblers looking for their own personal meccas.

The entire expanse of national forest and parklands around Panorama Point can be quite wet and chilly. Although the campground is only 800 feet in elevation, conditions are more representative of those higher up because the lake captures moisture-laden clouds that drift into its basin. Rainfall averages 40 inches in the lowlands, with up to 100 inches of snow recorded regularly at the highest points.

Lush vegetation is the result of all this moisture, and much of the land remains this way due to the extreme contours that have prevented loggers from getting at the plentiful bounty. Where loggers can't go, however, bugs can. A spruce beetle infestation set in a few years ago, and the forest is noticeably affected with browned, dreary limbs on the Engelmann spruce stands as you drive up the Baker Lake Road. Forest fires and selective thinning will eventually clear up the problem, but in the meantime, look forward to the views out over the lake from your campsite.

Campsites along the lake are best for privacy and proximity, but all sites are large and well spaced. The underbrush is surprisingly light, but with each site being luxuriously large, this is not a concern. Sites 5 and 6 are plum. On the loop, I would go for sites 9 or 10.

Don't confuse Panorama Point with Baker Lake Resort, a facility owned and operated by Puget Sound Energy that is just up the road from the Forest Service campground. In existence since the 1930s, Baker Lake Resort can be handy if you've forgotten supplies. You can buy groceries, rent a kayak, and even purchase a fishing license there.

## Panorama Point Campground

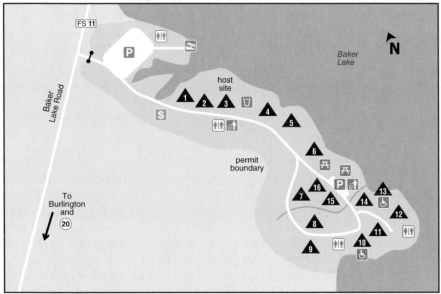

## GETTING THERE

From I-5 in Burlington, follow WA 20 east for approximately 22.5 miles to Baker Lake Road (FS 11). Head north on Baker Lake Road about 18 miles and follow the signs to the campground.

**GPS COORDINATES** N48° 43.207′ W121° 40.266′

# 27

# Silver Falls Campground

Beauty ★★★★ Privacy ★★★★★ Spaciousness ★★★★ Quiet ★★★★★ Security ★★★★ Cleanliness ★★★★

*The Lake Chelan area, while spectacularly beautiful, is overrun with tourists, but not far away lies this uncrowded, overlooked escape.*

This listing comes highly endorsed by a number of sources, including the manager of the state parks at Lake Chelan. That should tell you something.

In the summer, this third-deepest lake in the United States is a tourist and vacationer mecca for just about every variety of outdoor recreation you can imagine. Campgrounds overflow week after week.

This is not to take anything away from the spectacular beauty of the area. Unfortunately, this is the wry irony of so many spots in the Northwest. Their singular and stunning scenery is what attracts people to them. Sometimes the enthusiasm gets out of hand, as with Lake Chelan, in my opinion. If you can look beyond the cluster of lakeside resorts, condominiums, and RV parks marring the southern stretches of the shoreline, however, you'll see the natural splendor of a 55-mile-long, glacier-fed lake with forested mountain slopes rising as high as 8,000 feet.

Silver Falls Campground sits deep in the canyon-gouged Entiat River Valley in isolated splendor amid stands of cottonwood, pine, fir, and aspen. The Entiat River and Silver Creek

A fireplace at Silver Falls Campground

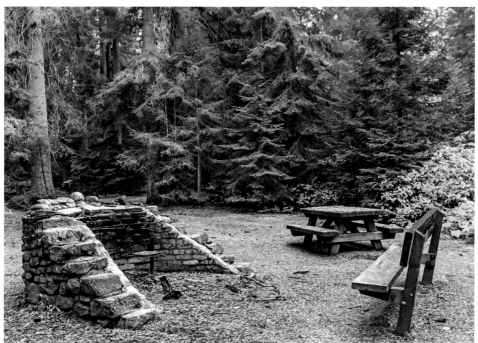

## KEY INFORMATION

**CONTACT:** 509-784-4700, fs.usda.gov
/recarea/okawen/recarea/?recid=58065

**OPEN:** Late May or early June–October,
depending on snow

**SITES:** 31 tent/trailer, 1 group (up to
60 people)

**EACH SITE HAS:** Picnic table, fire ring

**ASSIGNMENT:** First come, first served; group
reservations accepted at 877-444-6777 or
recreation.gov

**REGISTRATION:** Self-registration on-site,
online, or by phone

**AMENITIES:** Vault toilets, potable water

**PARKING:** In campground and at
individual sites

**FEE:** $12, $10 each additional vehicle,
$60 group site

**ELEVATION:** 2,437'

**RESTRICTIONS:**

**PETS:** On leash only

**FIRES:** Restricted during dry seasons

**ALCOHOL:** Permitted

**VEHICLES:** No ATVs in Okanogan-Wenatchee
National Forest

meet at the campground, and a trail leads 0.5 mile to the base of lovely Silver Falls. Other trailheads into the Entiat and Chelan mountains are a short drive from the campground. At road's end (nearly 40 miles from the main highway) is another Forest Service campground and a trailhead into the wild and remote southern portions of Glacier Peak Wilderness. This is terrain for experienced backpackers only because it has steep, grueling ascents over trails of crumbling, ancient, volcanic rock. At least half a dozen peaks above Entiat Meadows are in the 7,000- to 8,000-foot range. This is the eastern edge of the Cascade Mountains, where vegetation is not as dense as on the western side. Trails often traverse dry, sun-parched routes. Carry water from midsummer on, and be aware that thunderstorms can be sudden and fierce.

The landscape around Silver Falls is a contrast to the town below it, Entiat. Fed by a glacier of the same name, Entiat River and its innumerable small tributaries are part of the water supply for a small but thriving apple industry that got its start through the perseverance of a Caribbean farmer who settled in the Entiat Valley in 1868. His first attempts to cultivate peaches and plums failed miserably. He tried growing apples not long after, and the rest is history. The apple industry in Washington today is one of the state's most lucrative businesses.

Continuing deeper into the valley, one finds that the terraced orchards give way to the coolness of pine and cottonwood forests, with the grandeur of the rugged peaks providing a dramatic backdrop. Looking back, the rich blue-green of the Columbia, the lush assortment of fruit orchards on the benchlands, and the dry, rolling wheat fields of the eastern plateau at one glance reveal the diversity Washington offers travelers.

In addition to Silver Falls, Preston Falls and Entiat Falls are worthwhile side trips. Take a peek down into Box Canyon from the marked viewpoint. Mountain bikers will enjoy the network of Forest Service roads into the Entiat Valley, but remember that wheeled vehicles are not allowed in designated wilderness areas.

Those of you who can't resist the siren song of civilization nearby can sneak off to Lake Chelan, but don't go via FS 5900 (Shady Pass Road) even though a decent map might suggest that this is a good idea. It's longer to go back down Entiat Road, but trust the voice of experience on this one. Shady Pass Road can hardly be considered a road—more like a very bad wagon trail. Once, unknowing, I figured it for a shortcut to span the roughly 30 miles over the ridge to Lake Chelan. After traveling more than four hours over terrifyingly rutted and rock-laden roads and through the ghoulish remains of a very devastating forest fire in the full-on heat and dust of an August day, I arrived at Chelan's shore. Never did two cold beers taste so good! Never was I so happy to still have my muffler intact!

So if you must go, leave enough time and daylight to enjoy the views on the return. Coming out of Knapp Coulee on a velvety summer evening as the setting sun casts its glow over the Columbia River in rosy and golden hues is definitely one for the picture album.

## Silver Falls Campground

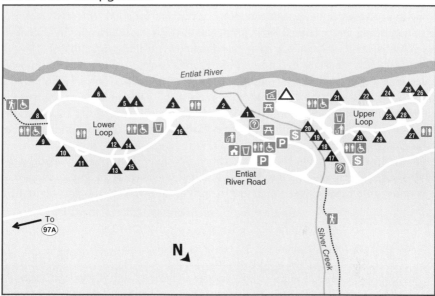

## GETTING THERE

From Wenatchee, drive north on US Alternate 97 about 15 miles to Entiat River Road (just south of the town of Entiat). Turn left (west) onto Entiat River Road (FS 51) and drive 30 miles to the campground.

**GPS COORDINATES** N47° 57.509'  W120° 32.200'

# 28

# Sulphur Creek Campground

Beauty ★★★★ Privacy ★★★★ Spaciousness ★★★★ Quiet ★★★★★ Security ★★★ Cleanliness ★★★★

*Here is a simple riverside campground in an almost forgotten area of Mount Baker–Snoqualmie National Forest.*

Sulphur Creek has come back to life. After being closed for over a decade due to flood damage, this campground (and its neighbor up the road, Buck Creek) is now accepting campers. The floods of 2003 were record-breaking in their damage along Suiattle Road. While repairs were being planned, disaster struck again. More intense flooding occurred in 2006, resulting in a washout and a landslide. It took out the road for good. This stretch of Mount Baker–Snoqualmie, and Suiattle Road in particular—which was the Pacific Crest Trail's only access point between I-90 and WA 20—was classified as off-limits indefinitely.

But those dark times are behind us now, thanks to years of advocacy from several organizations and individuals, including the Swinomish Indian Tribal Community and Washington Trails Association. The new road is gravel but just fine to drive at a reasonable speed. I'm a little ashamed to admit I almost overlooked this whole corridor because it's been closed for so long. A tip from a ranger pointed me in the right direction, and I'm so glad this campground is getting a second life.

Sulphur Creek is less than three hours from Seattle or Bellingham, making it a no-brainer for an easy getaway—far enough away that you're deep in the forest, and removed from your day-to-day, but close enough that the drive home won't be too difficult to manage

View of the Suiattle River from a campsite at Sulphur Creek Campground

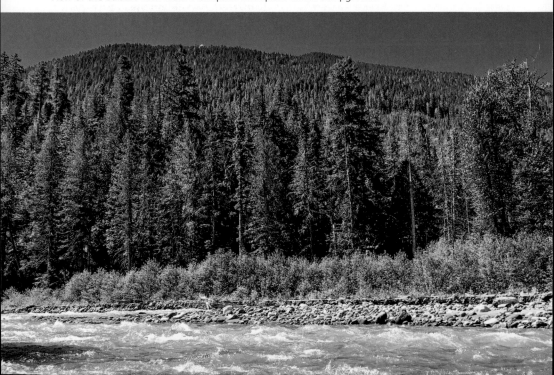

## KEY INFORMATION

**CONTACT:** 360-436-1155, Darrington Ranger Station, fs.usda.gov/recarea/mbs/recarea/?recid=62773

**OPEN:** Year-round

**SITES:** 17 (3 are double sites, up to 12 people, up to 2 vehicles)

**EACH SITE HAS:** Picnic table, tent pad, fire ring

**ASSIGNMENT:** First come, first served

**REGISTRATION:** Self-registration on-site

**AMENITIES:** Vault toilets, nonpotable water, no trash services

**PARKING:** At individual sites

**FEE:** $14 single, $25 group site, $7 each additional vehicle, $5 day use

**ELEVATION:** 1,584'

**RESTRICTIONS:**

**PETS:** On leash only

**FIRES:** In fire rings only

**ALCOHOL:** Permitted

**VEHICLES:** Large RVs and trailers not recommended

(if you live in the Seattle area, that is). Once you find yourself in this neck of the woods, it's the perfect small, primitive spot to enjoy old-growth Douglas-firs and set up a base for hiking. Suiattle River and Sulphur Creek frame the campground, and each site has no shortage of the sound of rushing water.

There isn't potable water here, so bring your own or be prepared to filter or boil. And, you guessed it, vault toilets. Bring supplies and you'll be just fine to kick back here in the simplicity of it all. Settle on site 8 or 9 if they're open because of their waterfront views, but each of the sites feels like a cozy sanctuary under the tall trees. The Suiattle River is glacier fed and not good for swimming (both because of the temperature and the current) but is a beautiful natural feature to admire from your hammock—if you can find a good spot to hang it. The river rolling by has an aqua hue, and the trees at its edges stretch up with bright green branches in early spring. Most of the campground is shady, and temperatures stay moderate in the area, so bring extra layers and firewood to make your nights as comfortable as possible. The camp hosts who keep an eye on Sulphur Creek are stationed up the road at Buck Creek Campground (page 79).

Because the road to get here was closed for over a decade, many of the area's trails haven't been well-trodden. Yes, folks, they're yours to frolic on for the first time ever! But in all seriousness, the trails this deep in an area that was off-limits for so many years may not be as well maintained as you're used to. Certainly a lot of work was put in to reopen them, but it will take a few more years—and a lot of footsteps—to make them look as well used as other hikes. I recommend a stop at the ranger station in Darrington to ask for advice and directions if you haven't already consulted the WTA website (wta.org) before leaving home. If the faint smell of Sulphur in the air makes you yearn for a quick soak, there is a piped warm spring nearby. Take the Sulphur Creek Trail for a 3.6-mile round-trip hike. The trail is neither well marked nor well traveled. The pool you'll find is small (seats two people) and not so much hot as it is pleasantly warm (at around 90°F), but you might deem it worth the steep climb through tangled growth (hint: veer left at the first fork and start climbing). If you can even find it, the pool takes about 20 minutes to fill after you sweep up the debris and open the pipe.

Other nearby trails include Downey Creek, the Suiattle Trail, and Green Mountain. Summer might provide you with berries and autumn with colors. Both the trail access and road access offer many options with diverse destinations for hikers and campers. At the time of writing this book, the trails have been open for just two seasons. Hopefully they'll stay quaint and peaceful but available to anyone willing to drive into this almost-forgotten area of the national forest.

## Sulphur Creek Campground

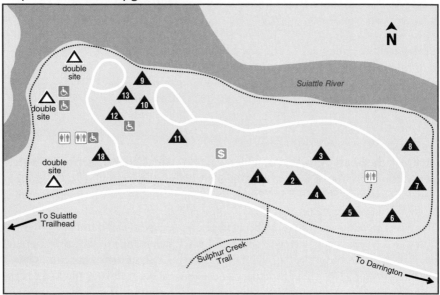

## GETTING THERE

From Darrington, head north on WA 530 about 7 miles. Turn right onto FS 26/Suiattle River Road. The campground will be on the right after 22 miles. Be aware that the road is gravel for the last stretch.

**GPS COORDINATES** N48° 14.907' W121° 11.673'

# CENTRAL CASCADES AND ENVIRONS

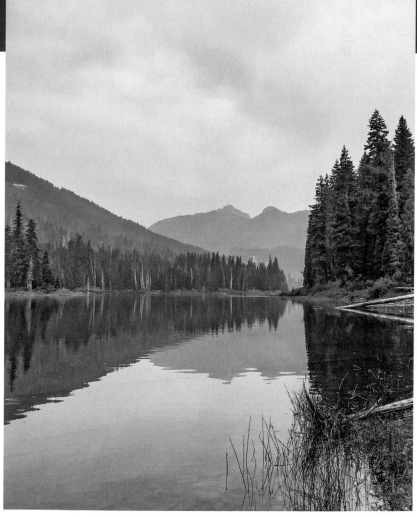

Cooper Lake at Owhi Campground (see page 110)

# 29

# Beckler River Campground

Beauty ★★★★ Privacy ★★★ Spaciousness ★★★ Quiet ★★★★ Security ★★★★★ Cleanliness ★★★★

*If you want a good base camp from which to hike ridges, run rivers, enjoy hot springs and historic towns, and day-trip into wilderness areas both north and south, Beckler is a great choice.*

You've started the day with a plan to leave Everett in the morning and be in Leavenworth in time for dinner by the campstove. By the time you pack the car, stop for coffee and pastries, crawl through the growing congestion of Snohomish, Monroe, Sultan, Startup, and Gold Bar (beware the speed traps in these hamlets of 25-miles-per-hour zones), gawk at Mount Index, take a short leg-stretching hike to Sunset Falls, and pause to watch kayakers as they thread the boulder gardens along the Skykomish River, it's clear you won't have much daylight left to enjoy the sights, sounds, and tastes of Leavenworth. Might as well find a campground close by!

Behold Beckler River—just when you need it! This is one of the few campgrounds along US 2 between Gold Bar and Leavenworth (much of US 2 can be aggravatingly slow going because it's a winding, two-lane road where passing is dangerous). Only 60 miles from Seattle, Beckler sits on the banks of the clear-running Beckler River 3 miles northeast of the historic village of Skykomish.

A heavy canopy of western Washington foliage shades the area around the campground as well as the numerous steep-sided river and creek valleys whose tributaries drain into the

The campground sits on the banks of clear-running Beckler River.

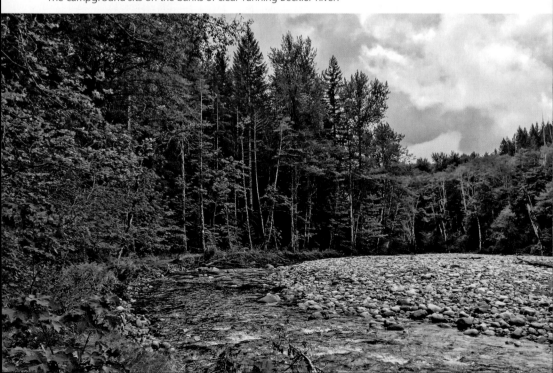

## KEY INFORMATION

**CONTACT:** 360-677-2414, Skykomish Ranger Station, tinyurl.com/beckler rivercampground

**OPEN:** Memorial Day weekend– mid-September, weather permitting

**SITES:** 27

**EACH SITE HAS:** Picnic table, fire pit with grill

**ASSIGNMENT:** First come, first served, or by reservation at 877-444-6777 or recreation.gov

**REGISTRATION:** Self-registration on-site, online, or by phone

**AMENITIES:** Vault toilets, potable water, trash services

**PARKING:** At individual sites

**FEE:** $16 single, $30 double, $8 each additional vehicle

**ELEVATION:** 1,085'

---

**RESTRICTIONS:**

**PETS:** On leash only

**QUIET HOURS:** From 10 p.m.–8 a.m.

**FIRES:** In fire pits only

**ALCOHOL:** Permitted

**VEHICLES:** Trailers and RVs up to 21'

Beckler River. The moist climate produces tall stands of Douglas-fir, western red cedar, oak, maple, and alder. At lower elevations, ferns and Oregon grape grow thick, while red and blue huckleberries can be found higher up. It's common to find skunk cabbage and trillium along the rivers. When I visited the campground, a mushroom-hunting club was having great success quickly filling their baskets with a wide assortment of delectable fungi (and perhaps a few not-so-delectable ones as well).

The absolute best sites are along the river—4, 6, 8, and 10. The next best are 26 and 27, these being on the river side of the loop. After this, it's a toss-up because they're all comparable in size (huge) and privacy (respectable). If you don't have to choose 1, 2, or 3, you will not have much to complain about. Sites 1–3 are less private and right near the entrance. Then again, you'll be next to knowledgeable camp hosts and close to a restroom, river access, and a trailhead.

Geologically, this area has a wonderment of sharply thrusting young granite pushing up through old, decomposed, and metamorphosed material. Estimates date the old rock as far back as 200 million years. A convenient place to view this clash of old and ancient is about 3 miles east of Skykomish where the Beckler Peak batholith crosses US 2. This is very close to the Straight Creek fault, which is used by geologists as the official dividing line between the eastern and western slopes of the Cascade Range.

A bit farther east is Stevens Pass, a popular ski resort in the wintertime. Once snowmelt clears the trails in summer (usually by mid-July), it's the place to catch the Pacific Crest Trail either north or south. East to west, Stevens Pass was the route of the Great Northern Railway when it was established in the 1890s by James T. Hill. Today, the Stevens Pass Historic District preserves what's left of the track and allows visitors to explore along it. A modern railway built to parallel the old route has a significance of its own as the longest railroad tunnel (8 miles) in the Western Hemisphere.

Trips into the Beckler backcountry should be preceded by a visit to the Skykomish Ranger Station. Heavy snow often keeps trails blocked longer than one would imagine. With all the high-quality mountain terrain to traverse, it may be tempting to strike out for the nearest ridge.

Henry M. Jackson Wilderness (named for a former Washington senator) lies to the north. Its 49 miles of hiking trails were once the cross-Cascade routes used by Native Americans and later by exploration teams. Follow the Forest Service road past Garland Hot Springs to reach the trailheads.

To the south is Alpine Lakes Wilderness—roughly 300,000 acres of high-altitude meadowlands and lake basins that are beloved by metropolitan Puget Sounders. In an effort to control the throngs into this extremely fragile area, the Forest Service has instituted a permit system that affects even day hikers. Now you can't say you didn't know. Trailheads into Alpine Lakes Wilderness are just west of Skykomish on Miller River Road, which becomes FS 6412.

## Beckler River Campground

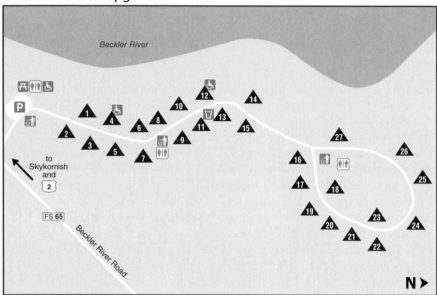

## GETTING THERE

From Skykomish, drive 1 mile east on US 2, turn left onto FS 65 (Beckler River Road), and drive 2 miles to the campground entrance on the left.

**GPS COORDINATES** N47° 44.075' W121° 19.942'

# 30

# △ Bedal Campground

Beauty ★★★★ Privacy ★★★★★ Spaciousness ★★★★★ Quiet ★★★★★ Security ★★★ Cleanliness ★★★★★

*This classic riverside setting remains unspoiled despite its proximity to a popular scenic loop drive.*

You've probably done what I've done—driven right by Bedal on the way to loftier destinations or while out for a day cruise of the Mountain Loop Scenic Byway.

It's easy to dismiss Bedal for its proximity to this busy scenic drive, a north–south connector within the Mount Baker–Snoqualmie National Forest. Hikers head east for deeper trail access points into Glacier Peak Wilderness. Mountain bikers churn toward Monte Cristo to the south. Fishers peel off at the White Chuck River to the north. Hedonists have heard about Kennedy Hot Springs and hope to partake of some debauchery. Families want the creature comforts of more-developed campgrounds in the Verlot stretch. RVers simply don't have enough elbow room or turning radius.

But for us tent campers, Bedal offers a classic riverside setting on the Sauk River unspoiled by the steady streams of passersby. Oddly enough, Mother Nature has been a source of chaos at Bedal, wreaking havoc in 2003 with torrential rains, slides, and high winds to the tune of $10 million in damage within the Mount Baker–Snoqualmie National Forest alone. With other windstorms following in 2006 and 2007, the Mountain Loop

Morning rays over the Adirondack shelter at site 18

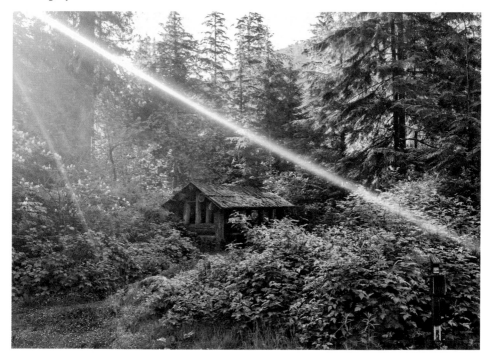

## KEY INFORMATION

**CONTACT:** 360-436-1155, Darrington Ranger Station; information on road and trail conditions (updated weekly) at fs.usda.gov/detail/mbs

**OPEN:** Memorial Day weekend–Labor Day weekend

**SITES:** 21

**EACH SITE HAS:** Picnic table, fire pit with grill

**ASSIGNMENT:** First come, first served, or by reservation for 13 of the sites, at 877-444-6777 or recreation.gov

**REGISTRATION:** Self-registration on-site, online, or by phone

**AMENITIES:** Vault toilets, no water, picnic shelter

**PARKING:** At individual sites

**FEE:** $14 single, $25 double, $7 each additional vehicle, $5 day use

**ELEVATION:** 1,300'

**RESTRICTIONS:**

**PETS:** On leash only

**FIRES:** In fire pits only

**ALCOHOL:** Permitted

**VEHICLES:** Trailers up to 21' (RVs not recommended)

---

Scenic Byway was closed until 2008 just south of Bedal, where a bridge went the way of many giant trees and tons of debris: downriver. Considering how close it is to some of the most dramatic washouts and its position along the silty banks of the Sauk, it's astounding that Bedal survived at all.

What a shame it would have been to lose this old friend of a campground. No information I found said one way or the other, but this must have been either a Civilian Conservation Corps (CCC) site or the work of miners who gave their hearts to this area more than a century ago. Reminiscent of the CCC era is a sturdy log shelter that is part of campsite 18. With its moss-coated roof and old-growth timber walls, it looks like it has weathered many a rough winter and probably even more rough-and-tumble visitors. The sense of history here gave me the odd but distinct sensation that I was being watched, if that's the right word to use. I've done a lot of solo road researching in the course of updating my books, but I've never experienced quite as eerie a sense of eyes on me as I did at Bedal. I'm not sure I felt threatened—more curious and slightly fascinated. It could simply have been the presence of the many huge old firs and cedars with their shaggy limbs and lichen drapery. Perhaps it was the shush, gurgle, slurp of the river as it slid quietly by. Perhaps it was the lack of a breeze on a heavy late-summer day. Maybe there are just enough glimpses of soaring mountain peaks to give one a sense of being looked down on. Whatever it was, there's a certain seductive quality in the air at Bedal, which, more than anything, is why I've included it here. I hope it will be part of your experience too.

Let me help you settle in quickly, and the choice of activity from there on out will be yours—everything from the aforementioned mountain biking to just-across-the-road trekking in Henry M. Jackson Wilderness. The campground is oval shaped, with two sites outside the entrance and several sites flanking either side of the camp road as you enter. Unless these are your only options, head for any of the sites along the Sauk River. Following the one-way road signs, these are in order as you make your way: 16, 15, 14, 13, 12. For ultimate privacy, go for site 7 (not on the river but tucked into a thick cluster of undergrowth). If the weather looks iffy, take site 18, and you can make money renting out the shelter for the night!

If you've come to Bedal for an extended stay, plan on at least one outing to Monte Cristo for the historical experience (check conditions here as well—floods have taken their toll, and rumor has it that vehicular travel is restricted). A second outing should take in some aspect of Glacier Peak Wilderness, due east as the crow flies but with trailheads possibly compromised by that nasty flood business. Pugh Mountain (within view of Bedal) may be an alternative and one that will give you a very good workout as well as stunning views.

## Bedal Campground

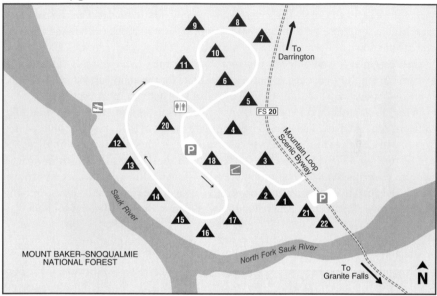

## GETTING THERE

From Darrington, drive south on Mountain Loop Scenic Byway (Forest Service Road 20) 18 miles. The campground entrance is on the right. The roadway turns to gravel at 4 miles.

**GPS COORDINATES** N48° 05.793' W121° 23.212'

# 31

# ⛺ Owhi Campground

Beauty ★★★★ Privacy ★★★★★ Spaciousness ★★★★★ Quiet ★★★★★ Security ★★★ Cleanliness ★★★★★

*Here's the ultimate tent camper's dream: a walk-in campground in an exquisite lakeside setting near alpine wilderness and the Pacific Crest Trail.*

If there is a tent camper's Shangri-la in Washington, it would have to be Owhi (pronounced OW-wee). It is, as far as I know, the largest walk-in-only (first-come, first-serve) car-camping campground in the entire state and, without a doubt, the most idyllic. The sites are not next to your car but down a short trail from the parking lot. You may have to walk 20-100 yards to find a site. Imagine yourself suddenly transported to a time when the tribes of the Columbia Valley came to the shores of deepest-blue Cooper Lake for the abundant fishing, well-stocked berry bushes, and tranquil setting in which to commune with mountain spirits.

Looking up at Chikamin Peak and Lemah Mountain—granite fortresses guarding the magnificent Alpine Lakes Wilderness just beyond the crest of their craggy profiles—one can easily relate to Chief Owhi, a prominent Yakima leader of the mid-1800s, whose passionate pursuit of the "good life" ended all too suddenly with the Treaty of 1855. Three years after agreeing to its terms but avoiding its application, Chief Owhi—who has been portrayed as having played a relatively passive and cooperative role in the remarkably unfair exchange of land from Native American to Anglo hands—was shot to death by federal soldiers.

Many sites at Owhi Campground are roomy enough for several tents.

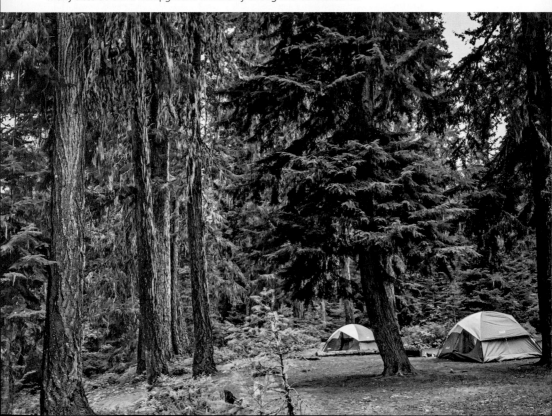

## KEY INFORMATION

**CONTACT:** 509-852-1100, tinyurl.com
/owhicampground

**OPEN:** Memorial Day (or later)–mid-October
(check with the Cle Elum Ranger District
509-852-1100 to confirm the roads and
campground are open)

**SITES:** 22

**EACH SITE HAS:** Picnic table, fire pit
with grill

**ASSIGNMENT:** First come, first served

**REGISTRATION:** Self-registration on-site

**AMENITIES:** Vault toilets, no water,
boat launch and dock, no trash service

**PARKING:** In general parking area

**FEE:** $14, $6 each additional vehicle

**ELEVATION:** 2,800'

---

**RESTRICTIONS:**

**PETS:** On leash only

**FIRES:** In fire pits only

**ALCOHOL:** Permitted

**VEHICLES:** No trailer or pickup-and-
camper parking

The passing of Chief Owhi seemed to be the straw that broke the camel's back for Washington's Native Americans, who had aggressively opposed giving up their lands. Disillusioned and broken spirited, they did not protest when the treaty was ratified a year after Owhi died, and the forceful removal of Native Americans from their many thousands of acres of sacred land to cramped reservations began in earnest in Washington.

Here in the serene kingdom of Chief Owhi's namesake campground, your pick of any of the 22 sites is denied only by your inability to get there ahead of the pack. And that can be a tough assignment. The Cle Elum River Valley is less than three hours from Seattle, mostly by way of an interstate, which makes it an easy mark for weekend warriors. Being at the top of the valley helps separate Owhi campers from those who are content with the more developed Wish Poosh, Red Mountain, Cle Elum River, and Salmon La Sac Campgrounds, which you pass on the way in.

However, there's no denying that Owhi's proximity to some of the easier eastern-access routes into the wildly popular Alpine Lakes Wilderness is its major selling point. Several trails within a mile or two of Owhi—and one that leaves right from the campground—connect to the Pacific Crest Trail, another attraction that draws heavy crowds.

Despite all this, Owhi's primitive setup, the serenity of motorless travel on Cooper Lake, and the panoramic views right from your camp chair are incentive enough to leave the madness of the trail to the trampling throngs. If you happen to be at Owhi midweek and you're hiked out, you might feel a bit like an ostracized relative who wasn't invited to the family reunion. You could be all alone! In that event, pull out that novel you've been dying to delve into all summer or get out the sketch pad. There's life after Alpine Lakes, as it turns out.

Let's talk about the drill before an Alpine Lakes adventure now. A quick tour through the campground is essential on arrival at Owhi. The parking areas—split into two—are above the campsites (roughly 100–300 yards away). Just standing at the edge of a parking lot and trying to assess what's available will get you nowhere fast, mainly because there's too much undergrowth between you and the campsites to see anything. (The campsites are down somewhat steep trails and spread along the shore.) Plus, while you're standing there doing your poor imitation of a scout, someone else is claiming territory.

To get a feel for the variety of sites and fully appreciate how the campsites "interact," you really have to start at one end and work your way along the network of trails to the other.

As you'll see, some of the sites are almost unnoticeable behind dense foliage. Others flaunt themselves. Still others are not far enough off the main camp thoroughfare for my taste, and then there are the double sites that have already been claimed—by the family reunions.

Still, there are plenty of sites that will please. If these are not taken, I would choose one of the sites on the southern side (18–22). They are at the bottom of a fairly steep drop from the parking area on a narrow, switchbacking, rooted trail (even Shangri-la has its problems), and they tend to be a bit more off the beaten path.

Of course, if a lakeside site exists, do I need to tell you what to do? Try not to be too obvious about your good fortune, but set your tent up—now!

## Owhi Campground

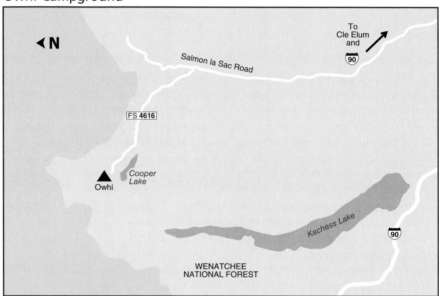

## GETTING THERE

From Roslyn, drive 19 miles north on WA 903 (Salmon la Sac Road). Turn left onto Forest Service Road 46, and go 5 miles to FS 4616. Turn right onto FS 4616, and continue 1 mile. Veer left onto Spur Road 113, and the campground is another 300 yards on the left.

**GPS COORDINATES** N47° 25.447' W121° 10.239'

# 32

# Rock Island Campground

Beauty ★★★★ Privacy ★★★★★ Spaciousness ★★★★★ Quiet ★★★★ Security ★★★ Cleanliness ★★★★★

*Explore Icicle Canyon, with its popular hiking and kayaking options, from this campground centered around the giant chunk of granite that is Rock Island.*

Ever heard of the "Rock Island Line"? Well, here's the campground personification of the railroad company that started as a one-track link and grew to control nearly all the lines in the Midwest. OK, so the comparison may be a stretch, but the name fits, and with all the spurs that lead off to interesting camping stations, it makes a good analogy.

Actually, the campground's name comes from the very obvious landmark plunked down in the middle of the stream just above the bridge: a gigantic chunk of granite broken off Grindstone Ridge that the creek is obliged to do-si-do around. Over eons the creek has cut quite deeply on either side of the rock, creating two narrow canyon gorges that send water shooting through in a constant, exhilarating roar. I was there in early fall after a desperately dry summer and found that even at low water levels, there's an impressive roar. It must be a wild scene during high runoff!

Four distinct "lines" now serve the Rock Island system, but it's easy to imagine that this campground probably had modest beginnings (just like the railroad company), with three innocent sites down by the creek—sites 1, 2, and 3. Let's call this loop A (although they are not designated as such). These sites sit quite exposed to the elements, mostly in full

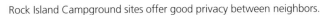

Rock Island Campground sites offer good privacy between neighbors.

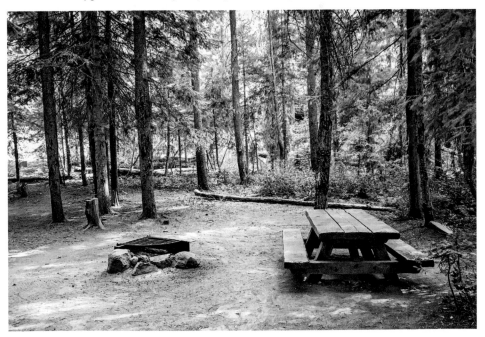

**CONTACT:** 509-548-2550, tinyurl.com /rockislandcampground

**OPEN:** May–October, weather permitting

**SITES:** 22

**EACH SITE HAS:** Picnic table, fire pit with grill

**ASSIGNMENT:** First come, first served

**REGISTRATION:** Self-registration on-site

**AMENITIES:** Vault toilets, well water, garbage service

**PARKING:** At individual sites

**FEE:** $18 single, $36 double, $10 each additional vehicle

**ELEVATION:** 2,900'

**RESTRICTIONS:**

**PETS:** On leash only

**FIRES:** In fire pits only

**ALCOHOL:** Permitted

**VEHICLES:** Trailers and RVs up to 22'

---

sunshine, and close enough to the edge of the creek bank that taking a giant step backward could find you among the rocks below. However, loop A has the only potable water I found, so it gets a gold star for that.

As the popularity of Icicle Canyon increased, a track pushed west, and loop B was born, with six sites (4–9) tripling the capacity. These take full advantage of the island view and are on a knoll of pillowy, half-shaded rocks. The summer sun up Icicle Canyon can be intense, so a little shade from ponderosas and firs is welcome. These are the best sites for drowning out incidental camp noise because they sit closest to the roaring surge around the "island."

Further westward expansion was inevitable, and more tracks were laid to accommodate settlement along loop C: sites 10–18. Timber has yet to be cleared in the hinterlands of loop C, so these sites are characterized by plenty of shade and generous undergrowth along low-bank stream frontage. I think I counted three vault toilets for nine tent sites, so the people-to-toilet odds are in your favor here.

A southern line came at last when funding allowed for a trestle (bridge) over the river. But the money soon ran out. Site 19 got the lion's share of space and sits in regal isolation above the creek in its own miniloop, looking down on the island across from loop B. Sites 20–22 would have to be considered weak attempts to continue the line (funding faltered), but they'll do if everything else is booked.

Rock Island may be at the end of the line for mechanized travel, but it's just the beginning of some glorious hiking options. This is the primary draw to Icicle Canyon (kayaking is probably second). To the north, south, and west lies Alpine Lakes Wilderness, acclaimed for the hundreds of places one may wander in high-country rapture even as the area desperately tries to hold up under the pressure that all its fame has put on its fragile ecosystems. Word of warning: I can't tell you not to go there (because everyone should have at least one Alpine Lakes notch on their hiking belt)—but the Forest Service can. They've had to establish a lottery system for visiting certain sections of the wilderness, so read up on the restrictions before you go at fs.fed.us/r6/wenatchee. This will save major disappointment at the end of a long journey.

If you happen to get denied access, never fear. Learn more about the geology and plant life of Icicle Creek with the scenic 4.5-mile loop trail that is a gentle walk along the banks of the creek, complete with interpretive signs. The official trailhead is at Chatter Creek, but you can pick it up at Rock Island and make the full loop from there.

Worth noting about the Icicle Creek area: forest fires nearly made this the end of the line for good in the past few years. You'll see evidence of the fire that threatened Leavenworth and Cashmere on the steep slopes above Icicle Creek. Be aware of fire-hazard levels and campfire restrictions at all times.

## Rock Island Campground

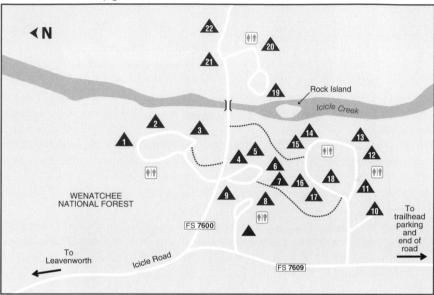

## GETTING THERE

From Leavenworth, take Icicle Road/Icicle Creek Road south and continue 18 miles (the road becomes Forest Service Road 7600 at about 8.25 miles). The campground will be on the left. Campsites are located in clusters on both sides of Icicle Creek and have their own access spur roads.

**GPS COORDINATES** N47° 36.424' W120° 55.071'

# 33

# Soda Springs Campground

Beauty ★★★★ Privacy ★★★★ Spaciousness ★★★★ Quiet ★★★★ Security ★★★ Cleanliness ★★★★★

*It's hard to imagine that this tiny, undeveloped spot was once sought out by droves of city dwellers who came to fill their jugs with its healing waters.*

From the ridiculous to the sublime. This is what you'll be thinking if you choose Soda Springs Campground as an alternative to Lake Wenatchee State Park.

While Lake Wenatchee State Park obviously has many glowing attributes (and has even made it into previous editions of this book), it's hardly the answer for anyone whose primary consideration in choosing a campground is seclusion. Lake Wenatchee State Park is where you go when you want a beautiful setting and are starved for companionship after a three-year stint on a deserted island.

On the other hand, Soda Springs is that deserted island. This is one of the tiniest, most undeveloped campgrounds you'll find in this book—and definitely within the sprawling 2.2 million acres of Wenatchee National Forest. The surprise is that only a few miles separate Soda Springs from Lake Wenatchee State Park, but the lake could easily be an ocean between the two.

Even more surprising is that Soda Springs was once sought out for the reputed health benefits of its waters. I haven't been able to substantiate this health claim with U.S. Forest Service

Even when it's full, Soda Springs is a remote getaway with only five campsites.

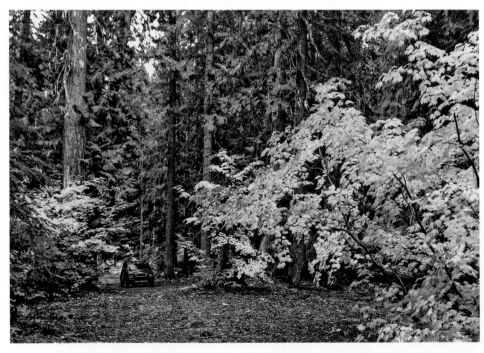

**CONTACT:** 509-763-3103, tinyurl.com
/sodaspringscampground

**OPEN:** May–October, weather permitting

**SITES:** 5

**EACH SITE HAS:** Picnic table, fire pit with grill

**ASSIGNMENT:** First come, first served

**REGISTRATION:** On-site

**AMENITIES:** Vault toilet, no water,
no garbage service

**PARKING:** At individual sites

**FEE:** None

**ELEVATION:** 2,000'

**RESTRICTIONS:**

**PETS:** On leash only

**FIRES:** In fire pits only

**ALCOHOL:** Permitted

**VEHICLES:** No RV turnaround
(sign at entrance)

personnel or history books, but a knowledgeable fellow hiker insisted that this was the place. I was having a hard time visualizing this pleasant but decidedly minuscule spot handling droves of jauntily clad day-trippers in their Model Ts speeding in from Seattle to fill their water jugs. If that scene were accurate, surely some enterprising opportunist, realizing his own personal manifest destiny, would have quickly slapped a health spa on the spot and charged admission.

Today, as you enter the campground (which has a NO TRAILER TURNAROUND sign prominently placed at the entrance), a well-worn log bench is the only obvious landmark showing where the foamy upwelling (that is, soda) makes its appearance as Soda Creek seeps downhill to find Little Wenatchee River. Otherwise, you'll find five very spare campsites indifferently dispersed, with one vault toilet, picnic tables, and fire pits being the only evidence that maybe someone else once washed ashore here.

Perhaps the better-kept secret of Soda Springs is found through the forest past campsite 3 on a sketchy path, over an ancient, fallen Douglas-fir giant (when that tree fell, it had to have been heard in Los Angeles), to the rocky outcropping overlooking a dramatic sweep of Little Wenatchee River. From here, Little Wenatchee River plummets into Little Wenatchee Falls and flows on as the headwaters of Lake Wenatchee, which is the source of Wenatchee River. It's hard to get away from the Wenatchee name around here.

Reflecting on the overkill of everything Wenatchee from this secret promontory, you're surrounded by the austere grandeur of true wilderness. In addition to the views below, there is a postcard scene to your left of a panorama of peaks that form the backbone of Nason Ridge. To your right is the eastern boundary of Henry M. Jackson Wilderness as it spills over into Wenatchee Basin. Behind you is the serpentine Wenatchee Ridge, known in literary hiking circles as Poet Ridge, which partially serves as the southeastern boundary of Glacier Peak Wilderness.

Long before these areas became protected wilderness lands, A. H. (Hal) Sylvester, the first Wenatchee National Forest superintendent, recognized that he had under his jurisdiction a whole lot of natural places that required names and he'd better come up with something a little more creative than Wenatchee. Fully up to the task, Sylvester set about mapping the region and handing out names to reflect his classical upbringing and love of poetry. As a result, we can thank Sylvester for Minotaur Lake, Theseus Lake, and Lake Valhalla in Henry M. Jackson Wilderness, and Poe Mountain, Irving Peak, Longfellow Mountain, Bryant Peak, and Whittier Peak in neighboring Glacier Peak Wilderness.

Nason Ridge Roadless Area, best known for its mountain goat population and a stupendous ridgetop ramble, missed out on the poetic names with more practical designations, such as Rock Mountain, Round Mountain, Mount Mastiff, Mount Howard, and Alpine Lookout. One of the few original fire lookouts in Wenatchee National Forest still in operation today, the structure hails from the Civilian Conservation Corps' heyday of the 1930s.

## Soda Springs Campground

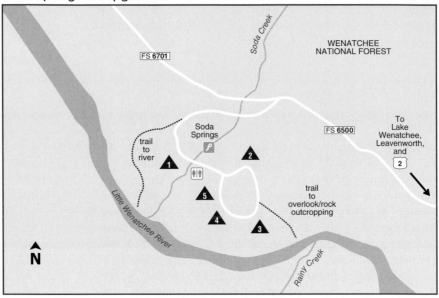

## GETTING THERE

From Leavenworth, drive west on US 2 to the Lake Wenatchee State Park turnoff (WA 207). Turn north and follow the road 12 miles. At the County Road 167 junction, veer west (left) onto Little Wenatchee River road. Turn right onto Forest Service Road 6500 and follow it 1.5 miles to the campground. Look for the NO TRAILER TURNAROUND sign at the entrance on the left. A campground has been built at Rainy Creek, but continue past this area about a mile.

**GPS COORDINATES** N47° 51.424' W120° 58.133'

# SOUTHERN
# CASCADES
# AND ENVIRONS

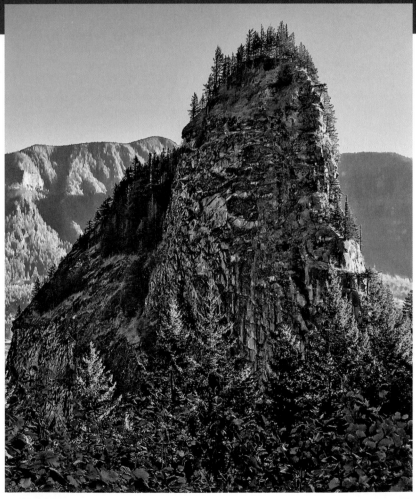

Beacon Rock offers a steep 2-mile round-trip hike to reach its 848-foot peak (see page 120).

# 34

# ⛺ Beacon Rock State Park Campground

Beauty ★★★★ Privacy ★★★★ Spaciousness ★★★★ Quiet ★★★★★ Security ★★★★ Cleanliness ★★★★★

*The Northwest's longest and largest river cutting a huge sea-level pass through the Cascade Mountains teams with the world's second-largest monolith to produce the main attractions at Beacon Rock State Park.*

Beacon Rock, once known as Castle Rock but renamed by Lewis and Clark in 1805, towers 848 feet above the mighty Columbia River in the Columbia River Gorge National Scenic Area and is second only to the Rock of Gibraltar in size. Several smaller but similar rock formations in this section of the gorge have prompted geologists to hypothesize that Beacon Rock may be the exposed volcanic plug of an ancient mountain, part of a range that preceded the Cascades. The monolith is estimated at 57,000 years old, actually young by geologic measure.

Apparently unimpressed by this massive adolescent of geologic time, the U.S. Army Corps of Engineers wanted to blast Beacon Rock to bits sometime around the turn of the century. Fortunately, railroad officials opposed the idea and stopped the demolition. Theirs wasn't a particularly noble reason, however. They simply didn't want rocks falling on their new tracks. Another popular idea at the time was to convert the rock into a commercial quarry.

The fate of Beacon Rock remained uncertain until 1915, when Henry Biddle bought it and proceeded to build a trail to its summit. The project cost him $15,000, a considerable sum in those days. When Biddle died, his heirs were instructed to sell Beacon Rock to the state of Washington for a mere dollar. One small restriction accompanied the low price, however. The land was to be preserved as a public park.

At first, Washington refused to honor the terms, so the Biddle family approached the state of Oregon with the same deal. An Oregon-owned park on Washington soil almost became a reality until Washington reconsidered and handed over the buck.

Visitors to Beacon Rock State Park Campground include weekenders from Portland, young couples testing their camping compatibility in a not-too-remote spot, and rock-climbers taking on Beacon Rock.

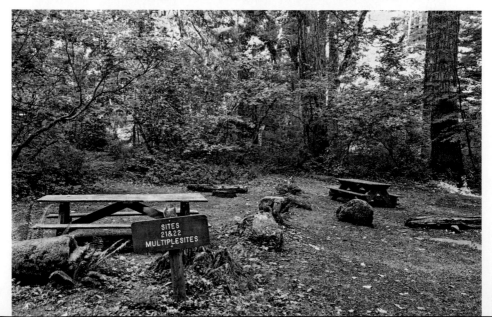

## KEY INFORMATION

**CONTACT:** 509-427-8265, Beacon Rock State Park; 360-902-8544, Washington State Parks; parks.state.wa.us

**OPEN:** Park, year-round; main campground, April 1–October 11; Woodard Creek and sites near moorage area, year-round

**SITES:** 28 standard at main campground; 5 with utilities, 2 primitive equestrian, and 2 moorage at Woodard Creek

**EACH SITE HAS:** Picnic table, fire pit with grill, shade trees

**ASSIGNMENT:** First come, first served, or by reservation at 888-CAMPOUT (888-226-7688)

**REGISTRATION:** Self-registration on-site or by phone

**AMENITIES:** Flush toilets, showers, dump station, playground, boat dock; picnic shelter and kitchen shelter at group site

**PARKING:** At individual sites, as marked for group site

**FEE:** $20–$45 standard and utility, $12 primitive

**ELEVATION:** 700'

---

**RESTRICTIONS:**

**PETS:** On leash only

**FIRES:** In fire pits when a burn ban is not in effect

**ALCOHOL:** Permitted

**VEHICLES:** A handful of sites accommodate RVs over 20'. The 5 utility sites on Woodard Creek allow for vehicles up to 40'.

Today, the trail that Henry built switchbacks a dizzying 52 times to the top and crosses 22 wooden bridges. Spectacular views up and down the gorge, including views of Oregon's Mount Hood and Washington's Mount Adams, are the reward.

Aside from Henry's mile-long piece of engineering (which is a must-see), you can follow a network of other paths throughout the park's interior to Rodney Falls and Hardy Falls. The Pacific Crest Trail intersects the park's trail system at the northeastern corner and takes the ambitious wanderer north out of the park and into steep terrain strewn with basaltic rubble to Table Mountain (3,419'). If you follow the Pacific Crest Trail south, you'll come to the point where it crosses into Oregon at a trailhead near the Bridge of the Gods (a worthwhile side trip of its own).

The hike to Hamilton Mountain (2,444') is a more doable distance for most hikers. Sitting beside Hardy Falls as it tumbles down Hardy Creek, with a forested mountain at your back, birds flitting, chipmunks scurrying, and fragrant wisps of campfire smoke wafting past, is as fine a Northwest outing as anyone can hope for.

As for camping options, the main campground is tucked against a forested hillside on the north side of WA 14. You get a taste of what lies ahead as you wind upward away from the river on the paved camp road under a thick canopy of tall trees. There are 28 sites cozily situated and generously spaced, all standard except for the first site as you enter the camp loop. This is the one primitive site, reserved for hikers and bikers. The main campground is accessible from early April to early October. In addition to the 28 standard sites, four more sites (two primitive equestrian and two moorage) are located down by the boat launch on the Columbia and are available all year. All sites are on a first-come, first-serve basis. I didn't notice any site that stood out from the others; they were equally appealing.

The good news is that the campground is primarily suited to tent campers, with narrow passage through the camp loop, a few tight turns, and limited clearance and parking discouraging the RVs—not to mention no hookups. As a result, Beacon Rock has an air of intimate detachment. There are travelers passing through—just stopping long enough to restore their road-weary bones by a roaring campfire. There are weekenders from Portland who have read about the glorious wildflower displays in the Hamilton Mountain meadows. There are young couples testing the camping compatibility factor in a spot not too remote. There are rock climbers who pit their skills against the face of Beacon Rock (except during the "no-climb" periods when the nesting raptors are not to be disturbed).

Whatever brings you to Beacon Rock, I hope you leave with the same feeling I had—that there should be more state parks with camping areas like this one. Even the parks system recognizes its own gem—Beacon Rock State Park ranked among the "best-kept secrets" on the Washington State Parks website. Go soon!

## GETTING THERE

From the junction with I-205 outside Vancouver, WA, drive east on WA 14 approximately 30 miles along the Columbia River. The campground entrance will be on your left past the state park sign and park office; Beacon Rock will be on your right.

**GPS COORDINATES** N45° 38.146' W122° 01.554'

The primitive campsite is reserved for hikers and bikers.

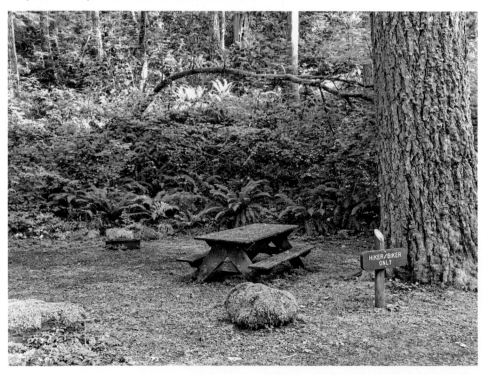

## Beacon Rock State Park Area

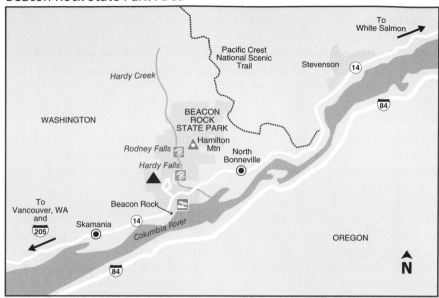

## Beacon Rock State Park Campground

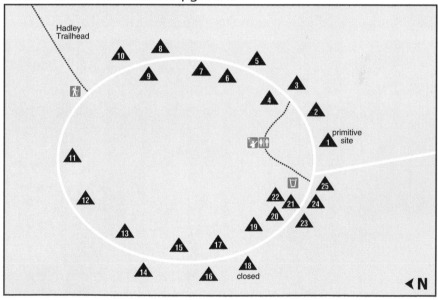

# 35

# ⚠ Goose Lake Campground

Beauty ★★★★ Privacy ★★★★ Spaciousness ★★★★★ Quiet ★★★★★ Security ★★★★ Cleanliness ★★★★

*Popular with anglers and hikers, this rustic campground is a tent camper's delight, particularly in fall, when the mosquitoes are fewer and huckleberries are plentiful.*

It would be cruel to lead you into the splendid alpine world of Indian Heaven Wilderness without giving you the bad news early on.

Just when the wildflowers burst into riotous displays of color, the snow has receded from all but the uppermost hiking trails, and daytime temperatures are warming to shirtsleeve conditions, an insidious presence prevails that is the nightmare of midsummer mountain trekkers throughout much of the Northwest. In a word, mosquitoes.

You laugh. "What are a few harmless bugs?" you ask.

Well, we're not talking about the occasional little devil that wanders into your tent just as you're about to doze off and decides to make a snack of your forehead. No, we're talking about droves. Swarms. Squadrons. Plague-sized packs. There's absolutely no relief from them when they're at their worst. Even a good insect repellent is often useless.

So, armed with this knowledge, you may decide to put Goose Lake Campground on your August and September list of places to visit. Besides fewer mosquitoes being in the higher altitudes at this time of year, there are bountiful huckleberries in late summer, and the scenery is certainly no less spectacular than in spring. Fall colors, for example, peak in late September.

Most of the sites here are tent-only, with only one large enough to accommodate an RV or trailer.

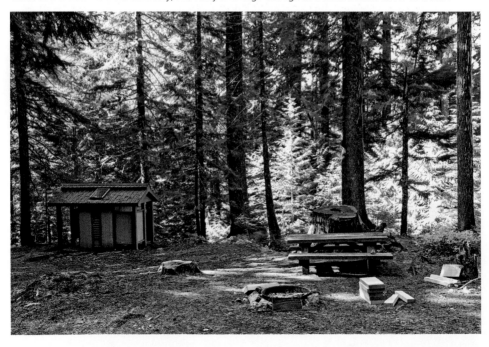

## KEY INFORMATION

**CONTACT:** 509-395-3400, tinyurl.com/gooselakecampground

**OPEN:** Mid-June–mid-September, depending on weather (visit in August and September to avoid the worst of the mosquitoes)

**SITES:** 18, mostly walk-in

**EACH SITE HAS:** Picnic table, fire pit with grill

**ASSIGNMENT:** First come, first served

**REGISTRATION:** On-site

**AMENITIES:** Vault toilets, no potable water, no hookups, boat ramp

**PARKING:** Near individual sites and in main parking area

**FEE:** $10, $5 each additional vehicle

**ELEVATION:** 3,143'

**RESTRICTIONS:**

**PETS:** On leash only

**FIRES:** In fire pits only

**ALCOHOL:** Permitted at campsite only

**VEHICLES:** Goose Lake has room for 1 trailer, up to 18'; RVs not recommended

Goose Lake Campground sits at almost 3,200 feet on Forest Service Road (FS) 6035 about 13 miles southwest of Trout Lake. The ranger station for the Mount Adams District of Gifford Pinchot National Forest is in Trout Lake. It manages the areas around Goose Lake, including Indian Heaven Wilderness and a strange area known as Big Lava Bed. It would be a good idea to pick up road maps, trail guides, and any of the other useful information at the ranger station to get the most out of your trip. The U.S. Forest Service system of roads in these parts is a tangle of spurs off the main routes and can easily lead to frustration if you get adventurous off the beaten path.

The campground is a tent camper's delight, with 18 tent sites and only one site large enough to accommodate a small RV or trailer, primarily because the access road is very narrow and doesn't lend itself to passage by large or wide vehicles.

It's been my experience that most camp loop roads are numbered counterclockwise, but Goose Lake chooses to be different. Site 1 is to the left as you enter the compound, and site 18 comes before site 17, for some reason, as you exit the loop. All sites have views of the lake and most are walk-in, as the parking area is well away from the actual campsite. Be aware that there is no potable water here.

The campground attracts mainly hikers and anglers. There is a boat ramp on the lake (for nonmotorized boats only), and regular stocking of rainbow trout means good eating over the campstove. If you want to pack it in, fish, then pack it out, it's worth knowing that many of the lakes in Indian Heaven Wilderness are planted with cutthroat trout. Check with the Department of Fish & Wildlife for any current fishing restrictions.

If your interests lean toward the archaeological, Indian Heaven is a unique place for study. This high, rolling bench area between volcanoes (explosive Mount St. Helens to the northwest and Mount Adams to the northeast) once attracted Native American tribes from as far away as Umatilla and Warm Springs in Oregon. Its 175 lakes, beautiful meadows, and abundant wildlife provided plenty of game, fish, and berries. The Native Americans also indulged in one of their favorite sports in an area now called the Indian Racetrack. Faint sections of the track are still evident along the southern boundary of the wilderness between Red Mountain and Berry Mountain.

Today, Indian Heaven is renowned for its huckleberry fields, and berry picking is zealously pursued by both natives and nonnatives. The Gifford Pinchot National Forest even maintains a "Huckleberry Hot Spots" page on its website. A 1932 agreement preserved a portion of the berry fields in Indian Heaven for Native American posterity, and signs indicate the reserved usage; be respectful of the tribes' berry rights.

For the geology buff, Goose Lake sits on the northern edge of the eerie Big Lava Bed. This scene resembles a moonscape. Early volcanic eruptions produced a lava flow that hardened more than 12,000 acres, leaving craters, caves, lava tubes, and other odd-shaped rock formations. The Forest Service warns that Big Lava Bed has few trails and is steep and rugged in places. If you bushwhack into the interior, keep in mind that the magnetic quality of the rock surrounding you can affect the accuracy of your compass. Toward Trout Lake, Ice Caves is another unusual volcanic formation worthy of exploration.

## Goose Lake Campground

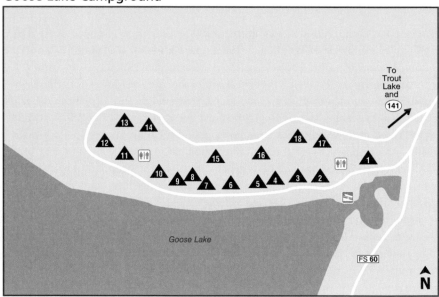

## GETTING THERE

From White Salmon on the Columbia River, drive north 22 miles on WA 141 to Trout Lake. Continue on WA 141 as it turns southwest and becomes FS 24 (Carson Guler Road) at about 5 miles. After another 2.5 miles, turn onto FS 60 and go approximately 5 miles to the campground.

**GPS COORDINATES** N45° 56.347' W121° 45.443'

# 36

# Lower Falls Campground

Beauty ★★★★ Privacy ★★★★ Spaciousness ★★★★★ Quiet ★★★★ Security ★★★ Cleanliness ★★★★★

*A good site for a base camp while you explore Mount St. Helens, this area also offers major waterfall viewing and lots of other outdoor activities.*

Not long after the 1980 eruption of Mount St. Helens, a small plane carried its umpteenth load of international news reporters and photographers on a media junket into the area of devastation. A local reporter familiar with the Northwest terrain was among the group. As the plane flew over vast tracts of gouged landscapes and treeless mountainsides, all except the local reporter gasped and swore softly at the destruction they witnessed below them. They took copious notes and jammed camera lenses up against the plane's windows, firing off numerous rounds of film with their motor drives.

Only the local reporter sat calmly and, at one point, quietly informed his comrades that they were a long way from the Mount St. Helens zone. What they saw below, he explained, were rather typical examples of a Northwest clear-cut. They may very well have been flying up the Lewis River Valley.

I've been back up the valley several times since first writing this entry, and the old clear-cuts are starting to fill in with a soft layer of younger trees. But I still like that story and I still think the best time to head for the Lower Falls Campground is about midnight on a moonless night. Now, it's not about shielding myself from the ugly clear-cutting. It's the only time

Lower Lewis River Falls

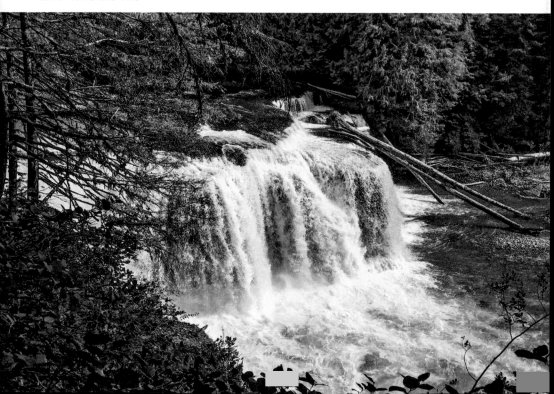

## KEY INFORMATION

**CONTACT:** 360-449-7800, fs.usda.gov
/giffordpinchot

**OPEN:** Memorial Day–October

**SITES:** 43

**EACH SITE HAS:** Picnic table, fire pit

**ASSIGNMENT:** First come, first served,
or by reservation at 877-444-6777 or visit
recreation.gov

**REGISTRATION:** Self-registration on-site

**AMENITIES:** Vault toilets, hand-pumped
water, firewood

**PARKING:** At individual sites

**FEE:** $15, $5 each additional vehicle

**ELEVATION:** 1,535'

**RESTRICTIONS:**

**PETS:** On leash only

**FIRES:** In fire pits only

**ALCOHOL:** Permitted

**VEHICLES:** RVs up to 60'

**OTHER:** Permits required for climbing
Mount St. Helens; check website for latest
information on volcanic activity, which
may prohibit climbing

---

I think that road is not full of either drivers not at all concerned about getting somewhere or drivers who are way too stressed about not getting somewhere fast enough!

Unfortunately, most of us don't want to find ourselves on a lonely stretch of backcountry roadway at midnight, so we're stuck behind each other for better or for worse. Enjoy what you can on the drive and look forward to getting to Lower Falls without undue stress. This is an area characterized by cloudy, damp weather, so if you're blessed with fewer clouds on the drive, you'll see Mount St. Helens at various points along the route. Some of the views are even marked. Take every opportunity you have to stop and enjoy them. Once at the falls, you'll be deep in the woods where views of mountain peaks disappear.

There in the forest the primary spectacle is a series of major waterfalls roaring off what are known geologically as "benches," wide tiers of rock formed over many thousands of years as glaciers; the Lewis River carved out the steep-sided V-shaped valley. The Forest Service has an extensive list of the waterfalls in the area, many of which are within an easy walk of Forest Service roads.

I have been to the lower of the three Lewis River Falls only at low-water times of the year—summer, to be exact. Much of the rock is exposed during low-runoff periods, but this makes for a totally different scene. The rock is worn smooth and polished, resembling a huge mass of flat-topped pillows. It's easy to imagine the thunderous splendor of these falls when water levels are high. Late spring would be the best time to see them in their glory.

Lower Falls Campground has undergone some renovation and features twice as many campsites as before. The original 20 are still the best because they're closer to the river and have more vegetation between them, providing the ultimate in privacy. Even the new sites have some undergrowth between them, making them an acceptable option as well. Unfortunately, the trend to accommodate RVs has affected Lower Falls, and sites can now handle rigs up to 60 feet long where once they were limited to a maximum of 20 feet. Ah, the good old days.

Keep in mind that this is a campground with few amenities—only one step up from primitive. Supplies are a long way back at Cougar (and they're limited even there), so plan to go in well prepared.

Activities in the Lewis River Valley—aside from waterfall viewing—include hiking, fishing, hunting, horse packing, canoeing, and volcano watching. There are endless trails in the neighborhood, some of which pass through the campground. The Lewis River Trail is a popular 13.6-mile, low-elevation meander. The river offers good trout and salmon catches at designated spots.

The Upper Lewis River canoe route can be a challenging 8 miles when heavy snowmelt turns some Class II stretches into Class IV. Check out the Mount St. Helens National Volcanic Monument Center in Swift if you're using the recreation area as a base camp to visit this modern-day geologic phenomenon. Give yourself several days just for Mount St. Helens. If you're interested in climbing the mountain, stop in at Jack's Restaurant on WA 503 west of Cougar for all the information (and permits) you'll need.

## Lower Falls Campground

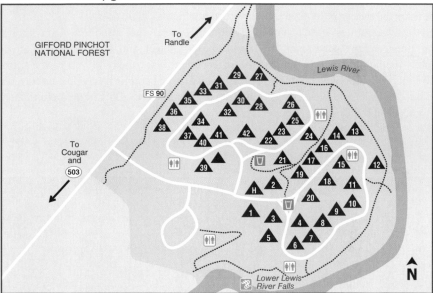

## GETTING THERE

Take the Woodland exit off I-5 (between Longview and Vancouver) and follow WA 503 (Lewis River Road) about 45 miles to Cougar. WA 503 beyond Cougar becomes FS 90. The campground is another 28 miles past Cougar on FS 90.

**GPS COORDINATES** N46° 09.380' W121° 52.975'

# 37

# Merrill Lake Campground

Beauty ★★★★ Privacy ★★★★ Spaciousness ★★★★★ Quiet ★★★★★ Security ★★ Cleanliness ★★★★

Primitive and remote, this campground south of Mount St. Helens lets you explore the area in relatively tourist-free solitude.

In May 1980 Mount St. Helens forever altered the landscape for miles around when it erupted and caused the worst natural disaster that western Washington is likely to see for a very long time. Only one other time in the recorded history of volcanic activity has a mountain exploded the way St. Helens did—more out of its side than its top. The St. Helens blast—500 times greater than the force of the atomic bomb at Hiroshima—spewed billions of tons of debris northward and created a fan-shaped path of destruction that stretched more than 150 square miles from northwest to northeast.

In the aftermath, St. Helens looked as if it had been savagely disemboweled with a giant scoop. Between the jagged south rim, lowered to 8,400 feet, and what was left of anything remotely mountainlike on the north rim, at 6,800 feet, were the remnants of the previous 9,677-foot peak. The view from the north showed a gaping amphitheater-like hollow, blackened beyond belief and measuring 1 mile wide by 2 miles long. Only hours before, this had been a scene of tranquil, snowcapped symmetry.

Nature trail at Merrill Lake Campground

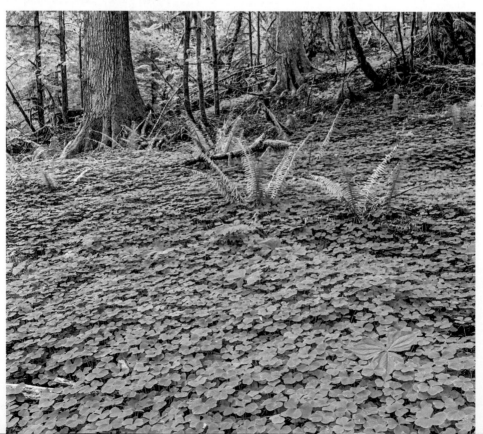

## KEY INFORMATION

**CONTACT:** 360-577-2025, fs.usda.gov
/giffordpinchot

**OPEN:** May 13–November 15

**SITES:** 8

**EACH SITE HAS:** Picnic table, fire pit with
grill, tent pads

**ASSIGNMENT:** First come, first served;
no reservations

**REGISTRATION:** Not necessary

**AMENITIES:** Vault toilets, potable water,
no trash service, boat launch

**PARKING:** At individual sites

**FEE:** None

**ELEVATION:** 1,650'

**RESTRICTIONS:**

**PETS:** On leash only

**FIRES:** In fire pits only

**ALCOHOL:** Permitted

**VEHICLES:** RVs prohibited

**OTHER:** Check the park's website for the
latest updates, including volcanic activity,
which may prohibit climbing.

Had Mount St. Helens chosen to send its pyroclastic plume in any other direction, it's highly doubtful that areas to the south, including the subject of this listing, would have been as remarkably untouched as they were. Aside from mudflows and flooding down the Kalama River, Lewis River, and Swift Creek watershed, these sections of federal- and state-managed lands sustained surprisingly little long-term damage.

In fact, campers who were enjoying the serene quiet of Merrill Lake on that fateful May morning must have been doing so with one eye nervously fixed in the direction of the mountain (which is roughly 6 air miles to the northeast). A "red zone" had recently been established for a 5-mile radius around the steaming crater, and only scientists and law enforcement officials were allowed inside it. When the mountain blew in 1980, those lucky enough to have chosen a weekend outing on the south side probably thought the plume of ash rising to an eventual height of 63,000 feet was the extent of the show. It wasn't until they returned home later that evening that television news reports showed them the full extent of the horror.

Today, four decades later, Merrill Lake Campground remains in wooded isolation just outside the boundaries of Gifford Pinchot National Forest and Mount St. Helens National Volcanic Monument. Recreational options around Merrill Lake include hiking on high- and lowland trails, boating, fishing, mountain biking, cross-country skiing, and caving.

The campground underwent a substantial face-lift after the flood of 1996, which gave the Department of Natural Resources (DNR) justification for addressing such needs as ADA compliance, adding new tent sites, upgrading existing sites, improving road conditions and the boat launch area, and making general cosmetic enhancements. Those who have had a love affair with Merrill Lake before will still be enamored of it. The same familiar rusticity, but better.

Just for the record, Merrill Lake is a favorite among DNR staff. That counts for a lot in my book!

In summer, most of the tourist throngs inundate Mount St. Helens from the north, leaving you to explore lands around the geologic wonder in relative solitude. Short drives up Forest Service roads lead to such interesting natural features as Ape Cave, a 2-mile lava tube that is representative of past volcanic activity. On the road to Ape Cave is the Trail of Two Forests, a self-interpretive walk over a 2,000-year-old lava bed. A short way up FS 24, which heads north from Lewis River Road at the east end of Swift Creek Reservoir, is the trailhead to Cedar Flats. This is a looped stroll through old-growth Douglas-fir in Cedar Flats Northern Research Natural Area. These are wintering grounds for Roosevelt elk.

If you're into some serious driving and want the best views of the Mount St. Helens devastation, take FS 25 north to its intersection with FS 99. This route takes you deep into the area of destruction to a viewpoint at Windy Ridge. These forest service roads are gravel, and sections are closed in winter. For full information on traveling either by foot or car in Mount St. Helens National Volcanic Monument, it's best to contact the park directly for current conditions. There is a park visitor center in Swift.

## Merrill Lake Campground

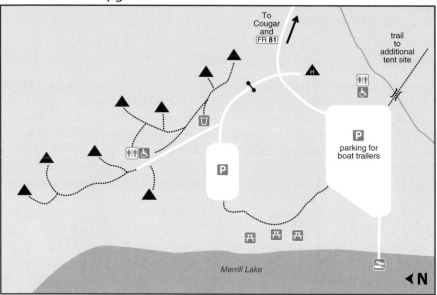

## GETTING THERE

Take Lewis River Road east from Woodland off I-5 to the small settlement of Cougar. Turn north, away from Yale Lake, onto FS 81, and travel 4.5 miles to the access road that leads to the campground.

**GPS COORDINATES** N46° 05.625'  W122° 19.199'

# 38

# Takhlakh Lake Campground

Beauty ★★★★★ Privacy ★★ Spaciousness ★★★ Quiet ★★★★★ Security ★★★★ Cleanliness ★★★★

There are many camping options in this lake-studded sector of Mount Adams's north-western flank, but none are quite as breathtaking as this when the mountain is in view. It's hard to get to, but it's worth it.

Just imagine: you're sitting in your campsite at Takhlakh Lake gazing out at a picture-perfect view of Mount Adams. It seems near enough that you could reach out with a paintbrush to add a little more white here, a little more blue there—a living canvas right at your fingertips.

If you've forgotten your paints, however, make sure you capture at least a photo or two of the scene. This is one of those spots that simply begs to be documented. On a calm and clear early morning, there can be two views of the mountain: the real-life one and the one mirrored in the lake. Definitely worth a frame or two.

There is no easy way to get to Takhlakh, which is part of its appeal and what makes it worthy of inclusion in this book. The confusing network of Forest Service roads can be downright irritating too if you don't have a good map of the area. I was beginning to feel like a rat in a maze after a while. It's a good idea to stop at the ranger station either in Randle to the north (the preferred route) or Trout Lake to the south. Pick up maps, trail information, and backcountry permits.

A campsite at Takhlakh Lake at the end of the season (mid-October)

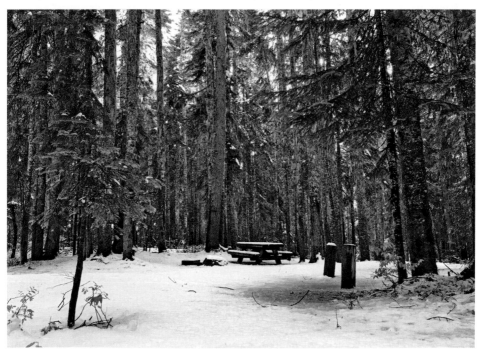

## KEY INFORMATION

**CONTACT:** 360-497-1100, tinyurl.com /takhlakh

**OPEN:** Mid-June–October, depending on snow

**SITES:** 54 (10 are tent only)

**EACH SITE HAS:** Picnic table, fire pit with grill

**ASSIGNMENT:** First come, first served; reservations accepted for 70% of sites July 1–October 31, at 877-444-6777 or recreation.gov

**REGISTRATION:** Self-registration on-site, online, and by phone

**AMENITIES:** Vault toilets, no water or hook-ups, trash collection, host, visitor center

**PARKING:** At individual sites and in walk-in parking area

**FEE:** $18 single, $30 double, $9 each additional vehicle

**ELEVATION:** 4,416'

---

### RESTRICTIONS:

**PETS:** Permitted

**FIRES:** In fire pits only; firewood for sale

**ALCOHOL:** Permitted

**VEHICLES:** Trailers and RVs up to 40'

**OTHER:** Nonmotorized boats only

---

Don't expect views of Mount Adams along the way to guide you. Except for a few stellar vistas across open farmlands as you head north from Trout Lake, say goodbye to the views until you're lakeside. These are the heavy alpine and subalpine timberlands of Gifford Pinchot National Forest. You don't want to spoil the surprise that awaits you at the lake, anyway. Besides, you'll be too busy making sure you're still on the right road (FS 23) as it wends its way through dense stands of trees, deceptively gaining altitude before reaching Takhlakh Lake at 4,400 feet.

Most of the 54 tent sites offer superb views of the lake and the mountain through stands of Douglas-fir, Engelmann spruce, pine, and subalpine fir. The main camping area is to the right as you drive in off the spur road from FS 23. These sites will be taken up quickly by RVs and trailers, but if you can find a spot lakeside and far enough off the loop, go for it. The camp host's post is prominently situated at the first site as you drive in, so if you have any questions, stop right there and ask.

An attractive new feature is the walk-in tenting section to the left as you come in off the spur road. There seemed to be more cars than there were campers, but it may be that the parking area is a bit small for the number of sites there—ten in all, numbered 45 through 54. They are fairly close together—I find this is a common practice with most tent-only areas. Do car campers seem more inclined to experience certain camaraderie in close quarters, or is it just a matter of available real estate? I wonder . . .

If you've come in search of lazy fishing opportunities, Takhlakh is a treat. Only nonmotorized boats are allowed on the glassy waters. With an Ansel Adams–like scene at your back, cast your line and wait for the trout lurking in the frigid glacial depths to find you.

For those with more ambitious recreational intentions, Mount Adams Wilderness is only minutes away. Trails lead ever higher as views of Washington's second-highest volcano get better and better with every step. Wildflowers carpet the higher meadows with bursts of color throughout late spring and early summer. Birds are plentiful and diverse. Wildlife runs the gamut of deer, marmots, squirrels, chipmunks, bobcats, elk, and moose.

A section of the Pacific Crest Trail passes Mount Adams on the western edge of the wilderness and is accessible from trailheads near Takhlakh. Climbers also use these routes to reach Mount Adams's summit. It's possible to use Takhlakh as a base camp for extended forays around Mount Adams on what is known as the Highline Trail. This is a rigorous navigation of 90% of the mountain. The last 10 percent would challenge even a mountain goat. Check with a ranger before tackling this.

While the spring and summer flower displays on Mount Adams can be inspiring, their loveliness is often offset by unwelcome visitors: mosquitoes. Although they vary from year to year, late summer and early fall are predictably the best times to avoid the pesky varmints altogether. I recommend the window between late August and early October for avoiding the crossfire (literally) of hunting season that follows soon after. Autumn colors make glorious photo opportunities in October, whereas huckleberry season usually peaks by late August.

## Takhlakh Lake Campground

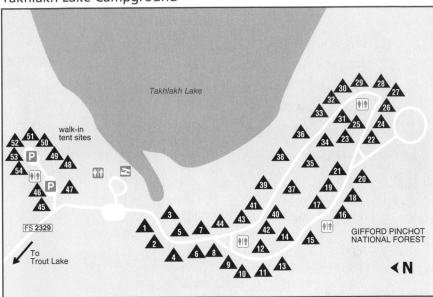

## GETTING THERE

Take CR 3 off WA 12 at Randle. Go south 2 miles to FS 23. After 29 miles, turn north onto FS 2329. The campground is a little over a mile in. To get there from Trout Lake, take FS 80 north to its intersection with FS 23. The campground is nearly the same distance as from Randle, but the road twists and turns and has vaguely marked intersections. The turnoff onto FS 2329 will be to the right coming from Trout Lake.

**GPS COORDINATES** N46° 16.896' W121° 35.947'

# NORTH CENTRAL WASHINGTON

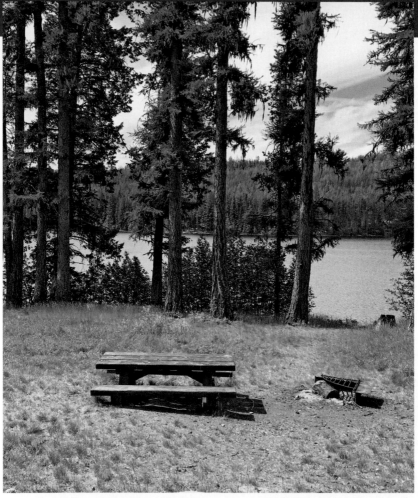

All the sites at Crawfish Lake Campground have views of the lake (see profile at right).

# 39

# Crawfish Lake Campground

Beauty ★★★★★ Privacy ★★★★ Spaciousness ★★★★★ Quiet ★★★★★ Security ★★★ Cleanliness ★★★★★

*This pretty spot is shared by campers, private landowners, and the Colville Indian Nation—and it's free!*

Here's one that has all the makings for being a fairly busy campground in the summer months, so you may want to put it on your agenda for when those still-warm days and crisp nights of autumn are upon us. Chances are good that you'll have the place to yourself.

Crawfish Lake is an odd mixed-use spot mainly because it has several different groups vying for its attention. On the northeastern shore are the campers enjoying their U.S. Forest Service campground with 19 very large and handsome tent sites, all of which have views of the lake, with about half the sites on its shoreline. The camp road enters the compound from the north side, allowing only sites 1, 2, and 3 to be placed around the loop at that end. The rest of the sites are staggered on either side of the camp road where it parallels the waterline and circles around a respectful distance from the reservation's boundary, giving sites 13 and 14 their fair share of space. A stand of ponderosa and larch serves as the natural buffer between federal and tribal lands—much more tasteful than an intrusive NO TRESPASSING sign might be. The conifers don't grow particularly thick here, but they balance the grassiness of the campsites. The general feel is one of openness and breeziness as the sun reflects brilliantly off the blue, blue water, sending a rich, radiant glow in all directions.

This site offers both a table and a bench for relaxing and taking in the views.

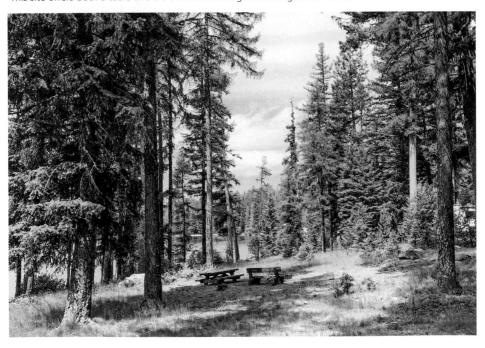

**CONTACT:** 509-486-2186, tinyurl.com/crawfishlake

**OPEN:** April–October, weather permitting

**SITES:** 19

**EACH SITE HAS:** Picnic table, fire pit with grill

**ASSIGNMENT:** First come, first served

**REGISTRATION:** Not necessary

**AMENITIES:** Vault toilets, nonpotable water, boat ramp, day-use area, no garbage service

**PARKING:** At individual sites

**FEE:** None

**ELEVATION:** 4,500'

**RESTRICTIONS:**

**PETS:** On leash only

**FIRES:** In fire pits only

**ALCOHOL:** Permitted

**VEHICLES:** Trailers and RVs up to 24' (tight turnarounds)

**OTHER:** Southern half of lake is within the Colville Indian Reservation, where special fishing and hunting permits are required.

On the far northwestern shore are the permanent homes and recreational cabins of private property owners, with manicured lawns down to the water's edge and personal boat docks. I'm sure they find the off-season the most enjoyable too. Best not to get too curious over there.

Halfway along the lake, the property changes to Native American ownership because Crawfish Lake has the unique honor of being split in two by the northern boundary of the Colville Indian Reservation. While there seems to be plenty of room for everyone to share in the lake's 80 acres of resources, the tribes have very specific regulations about fishing and hunting on their lands, so be as respectful of this as you would be of any private property owner if you plan to do some boating and/or fishing. Actually, you'll want to be more than respectful; the term is *law abiding*. You can be fined. For the most part, a state fishing license is all you need if you stay in the middle of the lake, but if you happen to fish from the shore within the reservation, you need a reservation license.

As a base camp for exploring all parts of the Okanogan highlands, lowlands, and benchlands in between, Crawfish Lake may not be the ideal choice. But then, the ideal choice won't have any camping spots available in the peak season! I've done my homework, and in all honesty, you'll be hard-pressed to find anything comparable to Crawfish Lake. Especially for the price: free. When you weigh all the other factors, there's nothing in the entire Okanogan camping inventory that offers what Crawfish Lake has: a great campsite; a decent-sized lake; easy access to the Okanogan's commercial zone (within 20 miles, all but the last couple of which are paved); a reasonable altitude; a highly scenic drive to and from; proximity to interesting byway and backway loops around Okanogan territory; and the blessing that it's in the opposite direction of where most of the camping crowd is headed.

Given that Crawfish Lake Campground's watery boundary backs up to a somewhat restrictive reservation, any land-based activities you plan to pursue will be mostly north and west of here. This means either backtracking down Forest Service Road (FS) 30 into the Tunk Valley (maybe stopping off at the Tunk Valley Wildlife Area) or staying north on FS 30 (also known as Peterson Road as it leaves Tunk Valley) to connect with Aeneas Valley Road. I have not driven them, but along the way to Aeneas Valley, the Chewiliken Road threads its way through the Chewiliken Valley and appears to offer an interesting day-tripping route in the immediate vicinity of Crawfish Lake. The Chewiliken Road skirts around the base of Tunk Mountain, which has an access road to a lookout on top.

I haven't been able to get a satisfactory answer on the background of Crawfish Lake's namesake inhabitants. Maybe you can. Yet another reason to make Crawfish Lake your Okanogan base. When was the last time you had crawfish étouffée on the campstove?

## Crawfish Lake Campground

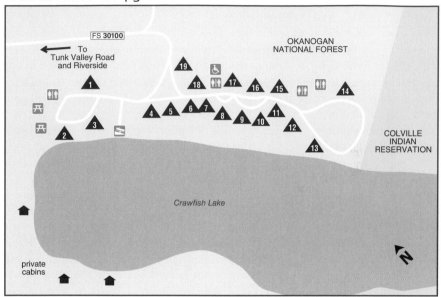

## GETTING THERE

From Riverside on US 97, go 18 miles east on County Road 9320 (Tunk Creek or Tunk Valley Road, depending on whom you ask), at which point the road becomes FS 30. Drive 2 miles, turn right onto spur 100, and the campground is less than 0.5 mile away. *Note:* Despite what you may see on various road maps or what you may read otherwise, this is the best way to find Crawfish Lake. Trust me on this one.

**GPS COORDINATES** N48° 29.084'  W119° 12.975'

# 40

# North Fork Nine Mile Campground

Beauty ★★★★★ Privacy ★★★ Spaciousness ★★★★★ Quiet ★★★★ Security ★★ Cleanliness ★★★

*This is a delightfully spacious and forested encampment in a land once cherished by Native Americans and exploited by miners.*

North Fork Nine Mile is to the western hills of the Okanogan Valley what Crawfish Lake is to the eastern plateau—a great base camp for exploring in just about every direction, whether by foot or by wheeled, motorized, or aquatic vehicle. In winter, strap on the cross-country skis or harness the malamute to the dogsled. This is an area as rich in Native American and pioneer lore as it is in outdoor adventure. Combining the two is a perfect way to uncover the secret haunts and hideouts of those who have passed this way and perhaps to create a few of your own.

Just down the road from Cold Springs but eminently more accessible, North Fork Nine Mile Camp—a delightfully spacious and wooded encampment within the boundaries of Loomis State Forest—is also governed by the Department of Natural Resources and offers the same amazing value as Cold Springs (that is, it's free).

Although it doesn't have Cold Springs' views or mountaintop perch, North Fork Nine Mile (at a respectable 3,500') does have hand-pumped water and high-bank real estate above North Fork Toats Coulee Creek. Go straight for site 5 and don't give it up—no matter how many gold nuggets or shots of whiskey someone may offer you. It's priceless! Of course, there is a slight drawback to site 5—found at the end of the loop drive, backing up to a steep embankment (to its right) and a creek down a steep embankment (to the left). There's not much room for error at site 5, so don't tell your enemies where you're headed, unless you have another escape route: the back door at site 5 is a mite tricky.

North Fork Nine Mile is an amazing value—free.

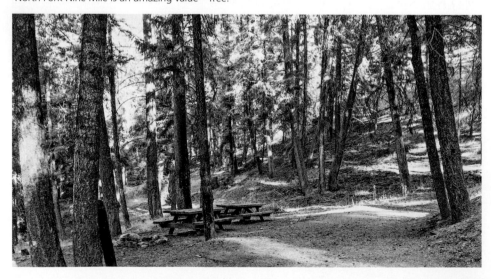

## KEY INFORMATION

**CONTACT:** 509-684-7474

**OPEN:** April 15–late November, weather permitting

**SITES:** 11

**EACH SITE HAS:** Picnic table, fire pit with grill

**ASSIGNMENT:** First come, first served

**REGISTRATION:** Not necessary

**AMENITIES:** Vault toilets, hand-pumped water

**PARKING:** At individual sites

**FEE:** None

**ELEVATION:** 3,500'

**RESTRICTIONS:**

**PETS:** On leash only

**FIRES:** In fire pits only

**ALCOHOL:** Permitted

**VEHICLES:** Trailers and RVs up to 20'

**OTHER:** All trash must be packed out.

---

About a hundred years ago, everybody around Toats Coulee had at least one enemy, and this was evidenced in some pretty bizarre and grisly goings-on. The Sinlahekin were the small, local tribe who claimed the lands of the narrow, namesake valley as their ancestral home. When gold was rumored to be plentiful "in them thar hills," every variety of opportunist descended on Loomis and the Sinlahekin, turning honest men into deranged schemers. Gold, silver, and copper were the main veins of luck pursued, and while no one got particularly rich, the Loomis area was a chaotic mix of miners, natives, and merchants as everyone gave it their best shot. Add to this the herders of the Phelps & Wadleigh cattle station and you've got the ingredients for a tough-living town. Hard to imagine when you drive through this tiny, clapboarded outpost that it was once the largest metropolis in Okanogan County.

The Sinlahekins had as their dubious leader Chief Sar-sarp-kin ("avalanche" in English), who boasted, boozed, and debauched his way around the Loomis and Toats Coulee lands in the last decades of the 19th century. Initially wary of the white man's intrusions, Chief Sar-sarp-kin came to be regarded as a mostly honorable native whose only fault, probably, was loving his homeland—and liquor—too much. In the end, having prevailed in entreating the federal government to allow his people to remain in Toats Coulee (rather than be shipped off to the Colville Reservation across the Okanogan River), he was done in at the hands of his own son (or so it is believed) over a family property dispute. Indeed, a sadly ironic end to the colorful chief's life. But bad luck followed him even into modern times: a massive 8-foot marble monument, erected at his gravesite by the Indian Department in 1912 mysteriously disappeared between 1972 and 1988 and has never been recovered. Nor does it seem that anyone can recall exactly when, during that time, it went missing.

Other enigmatic ghosts of the upper Sinlahekin include most of Chief Sar-sarp-kin's immediate (and large) family, several boomtown-era newspaper editors, Guy Waring—one of the area's first merchants (who eventually made permanent quarters over in the Methow), and Julius Loomis—the rich eccentric who was the "official" founder of Loomiston (as it was first known) and who was reported to have gone mad.

You'll go mad only trying to fit in all the fun things there are to do around Toats Coulee. Aside from stalking the history trail, you can enjoy beautiful, high Chopaka Lake Basin and take the opportunity to go fly-fishing (the only fishing allowed). The road up to Chopaka can test you, presenting the same conditions that confronted the pioneers, so be prepared for rough and steep.

Deer hunters populate the fields and forests of the Sinlahekin in the fall, as is evidenced by the deer-skinning stations at North Fork Nine Mile campsites. Don't let this deter you from a foray up into Pasayten Wilderness, where hunting is prohibited. The best access to Pasayten trails is at the Iron Gate trailhead on FS 500, which takes you quickly into broad meadows sweeping up to 8,000-foot peaks.

## North Fork Nine Mile Campground

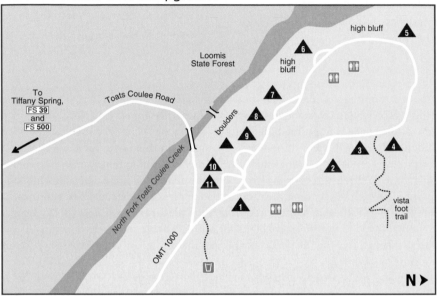

## GETTING THERE

From Loomis, go north 2 miles on the Loomis-Oroville Road. Turn left on Toats Coulee Road and stay on OMT 1000, passing its junction with OMT 2000, for 5.5 miles. Continue on OMT 1000 another 2.5 miles to the campground, the entrance to which is found just before the road turns sharply up to the left, crossing over North Fork Toats Coulee Creek.

**GPS COORDINATES** N48° 52.018'  W119° 46.193'

# NORTHEASTERN WASHINGTON

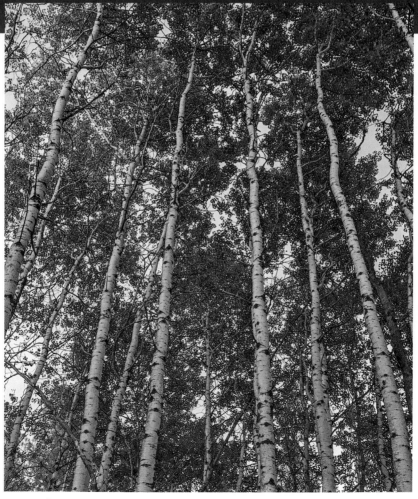

Aspens along a trail at Little Pend Oreille National Wildlife Refuge (see page 150)

# 41

# ⚠️ Ferry Lake Campground

Beauty ★★★★★ Privacy ★★★★ Spaciousness ★★★★★ Quiet ★★★★ Security ★★★ Cleanliness ★★★★

*This is camping for camping's sake . . . and maybe a little trout fishing and fossil finding.*

I've chosen Ferry Lake over Swan Lake as the place to camp along the Sanpoil River drainage south of Republic. Swan Lake has become the gathering point for the crowds, such as they are, out here. If you're going to come all this way to a place where camping is pretty much camping-simply-for-the-sake-of-camping and you're like me, you want as much solitude as you can find. Ferry Lake and the even smaller Long Lake are much better choices than Swan. So far, there's no formal campground at the dainty, picture-perfect Fish Lake.

In this extreme southwestern corner of the 1.1-million-acre Colville National Forest, lakes are stocked with brooks and rainbows, which makes fishing the main draw, after the old-fashioned whiling away your time in serene, forested settings. At Ferry Lake, the nine campsites are lined up along the lake, and it often seems as if the fish want to help you out by practically throwing themselves into the frying pan—they surface that close to the lake's edge, seemingly undisturbed by human presence.

Fishing is best in early spring and fall. Down at Long Lake, "fly-fishing only" is the rule, and all motors (even electric, which are allowed on Ferry Lake) are verboten. Anyone fishing must have a Washington fishing license, which can be purchased nearby in Republic.

The sites at Ferry Lake Campground have no shortage of water views.

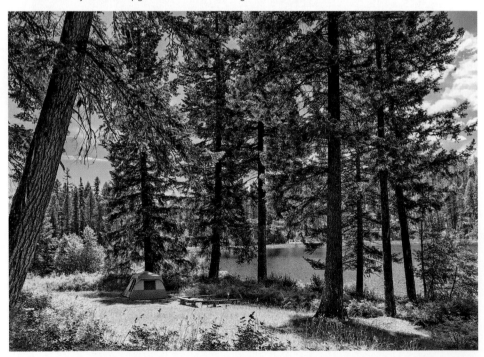

## KEY INFORMATION

**CONTACT:** 509-775-7400, fs.usda.gov
/recarea/colville/recarea/?recid=67866

**OPEN:** April–October, garbage collection
Memorial Day–Labor Day

**SITES:** 9; site 9 can serve as a group camp

**EACH SITE HAS:** Picnic table, fire pit and
grill; group site has large fire pit and
3 benches

**ASSIGNMENT:** First come, first served;
no reservations

**REGISTRATION:** On-site

**AMENITIES:** Vault toilets, no water, garbage
pickup with 3 garbage containers,
primitive boat ramp

**PARKING:** At individual sites

**FEE:** $6, $2 each additional vehicle

**ELEVATION:** 3,400'

---

**RESTRICTIONS:**

**PETS:** On leash only

**FIRES:** In fire pits only

**ALCOHOL:** Permitted at campsite

**VEHICLES:** Trailers and RVs up to 20'

**OTHER:** Fishing license required, no internal-
combustion boat engines on lake

Kids under age 15 don't need a license. Don't get caught fishing without a license or test the patience of the ranger by trying to pass as a 14-year-old.

If this means you end up in Republic for a license—and maybe a few camping supplies too—make a point of visiting the Stonerose Interpretive Center adjacent to the Republic Historical Center. Not only can you view ancient, amazing fossilized impressions of the plants, insects, and fish that lived in the area—and, apparently, nowhere else—nearly 50 million years ago, but for a fee, you can do your own digging and perhaps come home with your own Stonerose samples. The center allows people up to three fossils per person per day, but if you unearth something particularly noteworthy, they reserve the right to keep it. It's all in the name of scientific research. Maybe they'll name a rock after you, at least.

Evidence of previous activity around Ferry Lake is not quite as old as Stonerose fossils. The Civilian Conservation Corps hung around this territory back in the thirties and built, among many other structures, the one-of-a-kind kitchen shelter at Swan Lake that has become, intentionally or not, the epicenter of all campground activity. So if you've had your fill of isolated languishing over at Ferry Lake, take the trail between the two lakes (roughly 2 miles) and see what kind of action you can get in on at Swan—anything from an annual mountain biking festival to a private wedding (huckleberry canapé, anyone?). Technically part of the group site at Swan Lake, which accommodates up to 50 people, it's mostly just shelter from inclement weather. This is why you're camped at Ferry.

Before the Civilian Conservation Corps showed up, Native Americans used many parts of the Colville Forest's bountiful plant and berry harvests extensively for centuries. The campgrounds are essentially carved out of huckleberry patches shaded by larches, Douglas-firs, and ponderosa pines. Veteran pickers have been returning to this area for decades, a tradition fostered by Republic forest managers who occasionally burn portions of the area's understory to regenerate the berry bushes.

Aside from fishing and berry gathering, primary activities at Ferry Lake include hiking and mountain biking. The trail between Ferry and Swan lakes can be extended to include the 2.2-mile loop around Swan Lake as well. On foot, it takes a good day to get there and back to camp, but you'll still have time to park yourself by the lake and settle in for the loon calls at twilight. Most fat-tire enthusiasts will prefer to seek out more demanding routes, and there are 50 miles of them starting to appear on logging routes closed to motor vehicles. Popular routes go past beaver ponds—where the occasional moose can be found—and along Sheep Mountain and its views of the Kettle River Range.

Cool, wet weather prevails at Ferry Lake in the spring, whereas temperatures are generally very pleasant in the 70s or 80s in summer. Bugs are surprisingly not an issue here, and that could easily be the main reason you decide to seek out this relatively undiscovered part of Washington. Mosquitoes can be pesky in early summer, but with the kinds of summers we've had lately, their presence will be short-lived. A common annoyance elsewhere, biting flies are rarely a problem here.

## Ferry Lake Campground

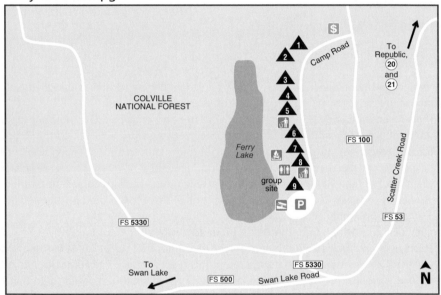

## GETTING THERE

From Republic on WA 20, drive 8.5 miles south on WA 21 along the Sanpoil River. Turn west on Scatter Creek Road (FS 53). Follow this paved road 6 miles. Turn north (right) on FS 5330 and go 1 mile, then head north again on FS 100 to the lake and campground.

**GPS COORDINATES** N48° 31.472' W118° 48.634'

# 42

# ⚠ Haag Cove Campground

Beauty ★★★★★ Privacy ★★★★ Spaciousness ★★★★★ Quiet ★★★★★ Security ★★★ Cleanliness ★★★★

*Here you'll find a 130-mile-long lake, mountains with the highest pass in Washington, and an abundant diversity of wildlife.*

Set on the western shore of Lake Roosevelt against the sprawling backdrop of Colville National Forest—a 1,095,368-acre parcel in central northeastern Washington—Haag Cove is one of 16 campgrounds within the magnificent Lake Roosevelt National Recreation Area, managed by the National Park Service.

Despite its proximity to Kettle Falls, the campground does not seem overrun and besieged the way so many of the other campgrounds in the recreation area are. The fact that it has no boat launch may be one reason why it gets less attention, because boating—mostly fast, mostly noisy—is a primary pastime of those who play within the recreation area.

I like it a lot for that reason. Plus, it's a very pretty and minimalist spot. The sites are well spaced, all have views of the lake and hillsides to the east, and there aren't enough of them to give one a sense of crowdedness. The best sites are on the south side (4–7), being large and close to the lake and having their own parking spaces. These will be grabbed by the RVers first, but don't feel obliged to leave them empty if you get first choice. Sites 10–18 are mainly walk-ins with a common parking area, but they're configured more intimately.

Campsites at Haag Cove have views of Lake Roosevelt.

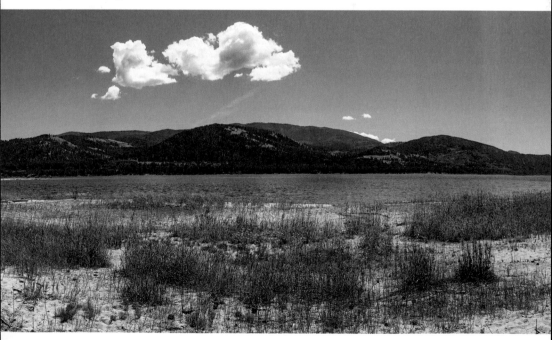

# KEY INFORMATION

**CONTACT:** 509-738-6366, nps.gov/laro

**OPEN:** Year-round

**SITES:** 16

**EACH SITE HAS:** Picnic table, fire pit with grill

**ASSIGNMENT:** First come, first served

**REGISTRATION:** On-site

**AMENITIES:** Vault toilets, water available seasonally, boat dock (no boat launch)

**PARKING:** At individual sites

**FEE:** $18 May–September, $9 October–April

**ELEVATION:** 1,305'

---

**RESTRICTIONS:**

**PETS:** On leash only

**FIRES:** In fire pits only

**ALCOHOL:** Permitted at campsite

**VEHICLES:** Trailers and RVs up to 26'

**OTHER:** Fishing license required, boat launch permit required

So, for maximum privacy, try for those closest to the lake. Leave the ones on the loop for latecomers who are happy to get a space at all.

The irony of Haag Cove's exquisite setting amid towering ponderosa pines and Douglas-firs is that its existence depends on a purely unnatural landmark. Lake Roosevelt was actually formed when the monolithic Grand Coulee Dam was built in 1941 to harness the free-flowing power of the Columbia River.

While you won't find the hundreds of salmon species that used to attract Native Americans to Kettle Falls, 30 other species of game fish make Lake Roosevelt a popular angling destination. You'll need a Washington license, which you can pick up at area marinas or hardware and sporting goods stores. If you're unfamiliar with the territory, you may want to stop at the visitor center in Kettle Falls for informative brochures and maps. Boats of every shape and size, motorized and nonmotorized, ply the waters of Lake Roosevelt. With 660 miles of shoreline, there's plenty of room for everyone. But if you plan to do some boating, be advised of the dos and don'ts on this particular body of water. The lake level varies according to the season. It's lowered as much as 100 feet in the wintertime, but walking the lake's exposed shoreline can make for an interesting outing.

Despite humankind's capricious rendering of the region's contours, this rugged, barren landscape gives one the sense of being in an unspoiled environment. Deep canyons, sagebrush hills, and forested mountains are home to many varieties of animal and bird populations. One of the best spots for observing and shooting—with a camera—is just north of Haag Cove in Sherman Creek Wildlife Area. Besides being a pretty area to explore, these 8,000 acres are safeguarded by the Washington Department of Fish and Wildlife, which protects the deer's winter habitat and the habitat of other mammals all year.

The confluence of Sherman Creek and Lake Roosevelt produces a high-quality fly-fishing spot. The only other campground in the vicinity is Sherman Creek. However, it's one of the few campgrounds in eastern Washington that's accessible only by boat.

Hiking options are plentiful and relatively uncrowded in Colville National Forest. Gentler terrain, a drier climate, and a longer season compared with the Cascades area make for ideal backcountry conditions. Sherman Pass, to the west on WA 20, is the high-altitude start (5,575') for trails north and south into the Kettle River Range. Across Lake Roosevelt to the east is Huckleberry Range. Call the Kettle Falls Ranger District (509-738-7700) for information.

Generally, the climate is warm and dry in summer, with daytime temperatures ranging between 75°F and 100°F. Temperatures drop to between 50°F and 60°F at night. Spring and fall are cooler but still dry and very pleasant. Eastern Washington winters vary but can often be cold and snowy. Since Haag Cove is open all year, check current weather conditions if you plan an off-season outing. Remember, Sherman Pass is the highest in the state and may prove impassable in bad weather.

A number of self-guided driving tours and scenic routes not far from Haag Cove offer another perspective of Grand Coulee Dam country. Bangs Mountain Loop, for example, takes you through stands of old-growth ponderosa pine. Historical points of interest at Fort Spokane and in Kettle Falls can be combined with a lovely drive on WA 25, which parallels Lake Roosevelt on the east side.

## Haag Cove Campground

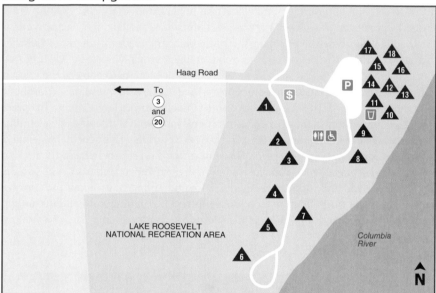

## GETTING THERE

From Kettle Falls (81 miles northwest of Spokane), drive west on WA 20 across the upper portion of the Columbia River. Stay on WA 20 as it turns south along the river to the turnoff for Inchelium–Kettle Falls Road (CR 3) at about 7 miles. Take Inchelium–Kettle Falls Road south 5 miles to the campground.

**GPS COORDINATES** N48° 33.683'  W118° 09.034'

# 43

#  Little Pend Oreille National Wildlife Refuge Campgrounds

Beauty ★★★★★ Privacy ★★★★ Spaciousness ★★★★ Quiet ★★★★ Security ★★★ Cleanliness ★★★★★

*If you can pronounce this one properly, you have lived in Washington for at least 10 years. But if you haven't been here yet, you're missing a state treasure!*

Let's get this out of the way. "Pond Oray." If you already know how to pronounce this unusual, French-sounding Native American name, you're either a Washington native or you've lived here at least a decade.

But if you've never been here, native or not, you're missing one of the supreme treasures of this state—a great opportunity for a wilderness adventure.

From the populated west side of the Cascades, the refuge should not be considered unless you have a full week to devote to getting there and being there. Just southeast of Colville and less than two hours north of Spokane, Little Pend Oreille National Wildlife Refuge (LPONWR) is a 40,200-acre tract on the western slope of the Selkirk Mountains and easily a good day's drive from Seattle. It has the distinction of being the only mountainous, mixed-conifer preserve in the United States (not including Alaska), with six distinct forest zones. The preserve is unquestionably worthy of the drive but is most enjoyable with a little advance planning.

And that's just the beginning of the superlatives describing this sanctuary, remarkable not only for its ongoing wildlife preservation and restoration efforts but also for the aura of serenity that seems to settle on you like a comforting blanket almost as soon as you arrive. It's a place where you find yourself whispering a lot and feeling guilty about the automobile noise. Driving faster than 10 miles per hour seems reckless. Going slowly induces a kind of reverence, in essence, with a bit of breathless anticipation thrown in.

A spacious campsite at Little Pend Oreille National Wildlife Refuge

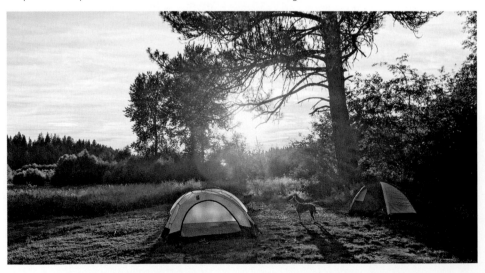

The campgrounds of the LPONWR are situated along what is termed the Wildlife Viewing Route on the refuge map. All are primitive, with fire rings, but they serve their purpose and don't intrude unnecessarily into the tranquil landscape. My favorite site is under the big tree at Potter's Pond. In addition to the campground campsites, designated sites are sprinkled throughout the refuge for use by hunters in the fall; there are about 31 of these dispersed sites, each marked with a carsonite post, available October 1–December 31.

Protecting the natural landscape was what motivated the early conservation movement that President Franklin Roosevelt supported when he signed the refuge into existence in 1939. Roosevelt created a total of 535 refuges, all so designated expressly to preserve vital wildlife habitats around the country. In the case of LPONWR, the purpose was to provide breeding grounds for migratory birds. Since its designation, the LPONWR has become an important management facility for an assortment of other wildlife as well.

Before it got protected status, the LPONWR hosted a variety of people who found compelling reasons of their own to inhabit the lands of the Little Pend Oreille. The first, of course, were transient Native Americans who used trails through the Little Pend Oreille Valley to reach the rich camas fields farther east and to socialize with other tribes at gathering points in the interior.

White man's exploration of the area was initiated by Canada's North West Company in the early 1800s not long after Lewis and Clark made their historic expedition west. Today the refuge still retains evidence of homesteading, logging, and mining activity that occurred around the turn of the 20th century. Some of the established campgrounds are the sites of former logging camps.

As you might imagine, birds are the focal point around the refuge. More than 180 species have been identified—from the regal bald eagle, who winters on the Little Pend Oreille River, to the warbling vireo, who makes its summer home on the refuge but flies south to Central America for the winter. The refuge maintains a checklist of birds known or anticipated to spend time there in any given season.

Bird-watching is followed in popularity by fishing. The refuge has three lakes, the Little Pend Oreille River, numerous tributaries, and an assortment of beaver ponds, which are open to those casting a line for catchable or catch-and-release fish throughout the fishing season. Two of the lakes are for fly-fishing only.

Wildlife viewing ranks at the top of my personal list of reasons to camp at LPONWR, and as I write this entry, I am mentally planning my trip back there soon. My only dilemma is choosing the best season. Spring lets loose the delightful songbirds and brings out the bears, and summer shows off colorful hummingbirds, the painted turtle, red-tailed hawks, and wild turkeys. (*Warning:* The mosquitoes are out in full force in early summer.) Fall gets into hunting season, a good time to stay away. Winter will find me camping at the nearest Colville motel but offers snowy perspectives on the snowshoe hare, pygmy owl, stealthy cougar, and furtive bobcat.

It's a tough call. I suppose I'll just have to ponder that one for a while . . .

## Little Pend Oreille National Wildlife Refuge Campgrounds

## GETTING THERE

From Colville, drive 6 miles east on WA 20. Turn right onto Artman-Gibson Road. At 1.7 miles (a four-way intersection), turn left onto Kitt-Narcisse Road and follow it 2.2 miles to the end of the pavement and a fork with two dirt roads. Bear right onto Bear Creek Road and drive 3.3 miles to the refuge headquarters. There's an information kiosk at the entrance to the headquarters.

**GPS COORDINATES** N48° 30.233' W117° 43.024'

# 44

# ⚠ Lyman Lake Campground

Beauty ★★★★★ Privacy ★★★★ Spaciousness ★★★★ Quiet ★★★★ Security ★★★ Cleanliness ★★★★★

*If you want small, secluded, and serene, you get it all in a ponderosa-pine forest in the remote southeastern corner of the Okanogan National Forest.*

As relatively easy as Lyman Lake is to find from Tonasket, you'd think this would be an immensely popular spot. Far from it. Therein lies the secret beauty of Lyman Lake. Everyone I asked knows about it, but no one really goes there. With some 200 high-mountain lakes and 400 at lower elevations around Okanogan country providing the most diverse options for fishing in the state, Lyman Lake is just enough off the beaten path to let you lose the crowds. And since I don't need fishing to define my outdoor experiences, I can enjoy Lyman for its other attributes.

Lyman Lake was truly off the beaten path for me—I got to it in a backdoor kind of way, relying on dumb luck, actually. I was on an extended road research trip and had already covered several hundred miles of the central Columbia River Basin by making a huge loop, starting in Lake Chelan on the morning of the first day and returning there on the night of the second. Don't try this if you're out to have a relaxing time or need your car to last several more years.

Lyman Lake Campground is primitive, small (with only four sites), free, and beautiful.

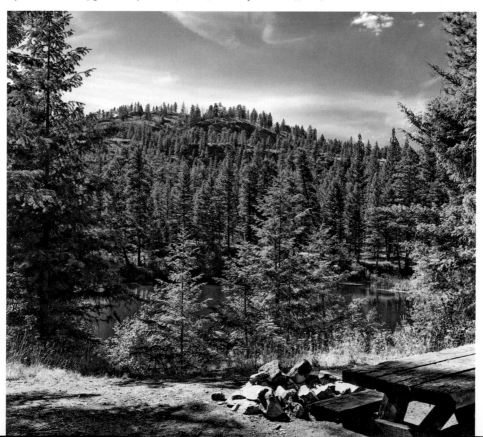

# KEY INFORMATION

**CONTACT:** 509-486-2186, tinyurl.com/lymanlakecampground

**OPEN:** June–September, weather permitting

**SITES:** 4

**EACH SITE HAS:** Picnic table, fire ring

**ASSIGNMENT:** First come, first served

**REGISTRATION:** On-site

**AMENITIES:** Vault toilet, no water, no garbage service

**PARKING:** At individual sites

**FEE:** None

**ELEVATION:** 2,900'

**RESTRICTIONS:**

**PETS:** On leash only

**FIRES:** In fire pits only

**ALCOHOL:** Permitted

**VEHICLES:** Trailers and RVs up to 24'

At any rate, after a delightful breeze through the Ferry Lake group, I was all for a short-cut to my next destination. I checked the map. Looked simple enough. West Sanpoil River Road. Well, I'm here to tell you that there is no "official" West Sanpoil River Road, just a goat track that masquerades as a U.S. Forest Service road on most maps. (You'll come to learn that this is common out here in the wilds of the Okanogan National Forest.)

Applying my best bushwhacking skills (in a car), I forged ahead, flattening old-growth weeds in my path (remorselessly), juddering across more cattle guards than I could count (methinks I have passed over a few too many to be going in the right direction), and crossing streambeds that didn't appear to have been disturbed since the last fur trappers skulked through. My perseverance and gut instinct paid off, and within several hours I burst out onto the edge of the beautiful Aeneas Valley. From there, I followed the signs to Lyman Lake. I was lucky. If you find yourself on the same track, save your car's undercarriage—go back and follow the directions at the end of this entry.

When I pulled in, a U.S. Forest Service ranger was just arriving as well. This I took as a very good sign. Although I was on the outer fringes of forest service jurisdiction and at the last public stop before venturing into the private reserve of the Colville Nation down the Lyman Lake–Moses Meadow Road, I found that Lyman was not outside Forest Service supervision radar after all.

However, there's not a whole lot to supervise. Lyman is only four sites, with one vault toilet. A no-frills kind of place. A dispersed camping area for hunters is around the far side of the lake, and a semblance of a boat launch (for hand-carried, nonmotorized boats only) is on the southern end.

Lyman is small only in the number of campsites, however, and I'm kind of glad that the Forest Service has not seen the need to add more. There's certainly plenty of room to do so. A long access road reveals much undeveloped land on either side, and the same goes for most of the area in the campground proper that's not a camping site per se. This makes for sites that are defined not by their proximity to each other but rather by how much space you feel you need to establish your claim. Each site sits with at least one boundary on Lyman Lake. The lake itself takes up only 4 acres, so the general sense (if you're not having to share with others) is that you've stumbled on a delightfully private little oasis.

If, like me, you're not much for fishing, the area around Lyman Lake is laced with trails that take you to high points above the valley floor for superb views. The Aeneas Valley makes for a great driving tour, with an Old West feeling to the ranch buildings dotting the broad pasturelands. A good loop trip for sampling the local terrain would combine Cape LaBelle Road, WA 20, and Aeneas Valley Road.

By the way, if you do fancy fishing at Lyman Lake, it's stocked with eastern brook trout, and I hear it's fantastic in the fall. But keep that to yourself.

## Lyman Lake Campground

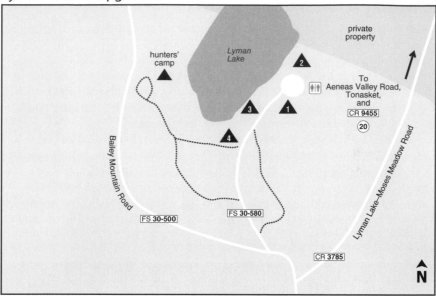

## GETTING THERE

From Tonasket, go 18 miles east on WA 20 to CR 9455 (Aeneas Valley Road). Turn right and drive 13 miles to CR 3785 (Lyman Lake–Moses Meadow Road). Turn right, and you'll see the campground 2.5 miles in on the right.

**GPS COORDINATES** N48° 31.265'  W119° 01.167'

# 45

# ⚠ Mount Spokane State Park:
## BALD KNOB CAMPGROUND

Beauty ★★★★ Privacy ★★★★ Spaciousness ★★★★ Quiet ★★★★★ Security ★★★★ Cleanliness ★★★★★

*Our largest state park has plenty of trails, majestic trees, and dazzling views of eastern Washington, Idaho, Montana, and Canada.*

You're lucky if you land one of the eight first-come, first-serve campsites on Mount Spokane. This is a no-frills seasonal campground with supreme access to trails and views.

Mount Spokane is the largest state park at nearly 14,000 acres, located just an hour northeast of Spokane. It was established as a state park in 1927 with just 1,500 acres. There's a lot of history prior to it entering the state park system; Native Americans hiked to the summit long before white settlers made their way to Spokane.

It's beautiful—it's beautiful when you're skiing or snowshoeing, when you're hiking, running a trail race, or picnicking. This cozy campground is technically known as Bald Knob, though most people seem to refer to it as Mount Spokane Campground. If you're already planning to camp in the area, take your chances and drive up to the loop. Worst case scenario: the campground is full and you get to drive to the summit, take in the

Mount Spokane State Park, with the larches beginning to turn

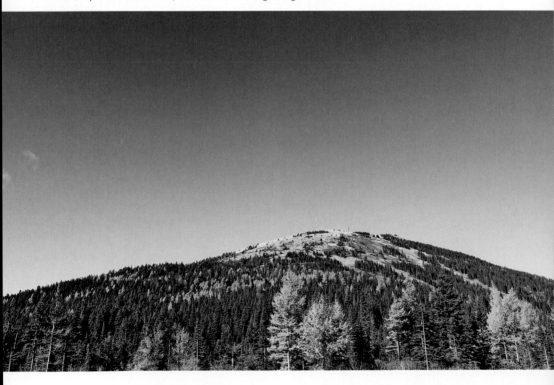

## KEY INFORMATION

**CONTACT:** 509-238-4258, mountspokane.org

**OPEN:** July 1–September 14, depending on snow conditions

**SITES:** 8

**EACH SITE HAS:** Picnic table, fire pit with grill

**ASSIGNMENT:** First come, first served

**REGISTRATION:** On-site

**AMENITIES:** Flush toilet, potable water, no garbage service

**PARKING:** At individual sites

**FEE:** $12

**ELEVATION:** 5,761'

**RESTRICTIONS:**

**PETS:** On leash only

**FIRES:** In fire pits only

**ALCOHOL:** Permitted

**VEHICLES:** Trailers and RVs up to 30', though not recommended (limited space)

---

scenery, maybe go for a hike, then head to Riverside State Park (see page 159) or somewhere else to spend the night.

The campsites admittedly aren't much to write home about—a fire pit, dirt, and a picnic table. A couple are slightly more private than the others. Even so, they're perfectly situated for surveying the mountain and its surroundings. But let's talk about the park.

If you hike up from the campground (you can take the road or hike the 3 miles using Trail 130 to Trail 140), at the summit you can explore the Vista House and take in the scenery at 5,883 feet. Look east into Idaho, where you'll get a peek of the Cabinet Mountains and lakes Pend Oreille and Coeur D'Alene. You can see Montana on a clear day. Look south to see where the Selkirk Mountains start and north toward the rest of the range making its way into Canada. Walk around to take in the view from all angles.

August is the perfect time to pick huckleberries, which are dotted across the mountain (there's a patch on Trail 140 on the way to the summit). Wildlife viewing is a nice way to pass the time while you hang out in the shade of a large old-growth tree. There are lots of birds to look out for as well—warblers, flycatchers, owls, nuthatches, thrushes, and woodpeckers, to name a few.

If you're a mountain biker, there are trails here for you as well—about 90 miles of them. Add to that 100 miles of horse trails and another 100 miles of hiking trails and you can see why this park delights so many. Visit the Friends of Mount Spokane State Park website listed in the Key Information for much more detailed maps and brochures. Once in a while you'll catch an interpreter out on a trail guiding summer hikes or winter snowshoeing.

Just a 2-minute walk from the campground is a covered picnic shelter with a wood-fire grill. This is a good spot for eating your meals in the shade. It's big and comfortable and used by many day hikers. South of Knob Hill is the fire lookout on Quartz Mountain, which is worth hiking over to. In its original location on Mount Spokane, it was repaired and rebuilt numerous times due mainly to damage each winter from icing. At some point, the DNR decided the lookout was costing more money than it was worth and planned to destroy it, but before demolition, the park asked to have it. The structure was relocated to its present day spot (after some years), and has been restored and maintained for use as a cabin. It's now available for rent if you need a glamping stay at this point in your travels. Better yet, get one of those eight campsites at Bald Knob.

## Mount Spokane State Park: Bald Knob Campground

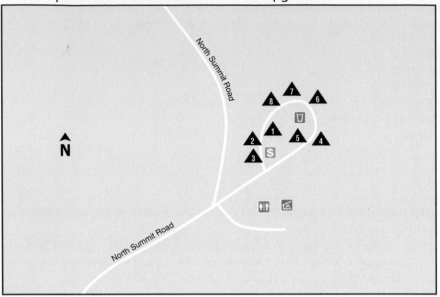

## GETTING THERE

From Spokane, take North Mount Spokane Park Drive (Mount Spokane Highway) to the park entrance. Continue on the road almost 3 miles and turn left on North Summit Road. The campground will be on your right.

**GPS COORDINATES** N47° 55.530'  W117° 06.763'

# 46

# ⚠ Riverside State Park Campgrounds

Beauty ★★★★ Privacy ★★★ Spaciousness ★★★★★ Quiet ★★★ Security ★★★★ Cleanliness ★★★★

*Land, trails, rocks, rivers, lakes, history—between these four campgrounds, Riverside has it all. It's a beautiful escape from a nearby urban center.*

No matter what kind of outdoor enthusiast you are, Riverside has you covered. Boating, rock climbing, hiking, biking, running, snowshoeing, and horseback riding are all possibilities here—it simply depends what kind of time you have, what the weather's like, and what you're in the mood for.

Riverside State Park, established in 1933, is situated along the Spokane and Little Spokane Rivers and boasts nearly 200,000 feet of shoreline. The park sits on more than 11,000 acres, making it the second-largest state park in Washington (behind Mount Spokane State Park). It includes lakes, marshes, wildlife, and trails—lots and lots of trails. It also has four distinct campgrounds.

Most of the park lies just outside the northwest border of the city of Spokane (aside from Bowl and Pitcher, which lines the western edge of town not far from Spokane Falls Community College). Everyone who lives in Spokane knows the park, even if they don't spend any time there. Some residents, however, make it a part of their daily lives with trail running

View of the Spokane River from Riverside State Park

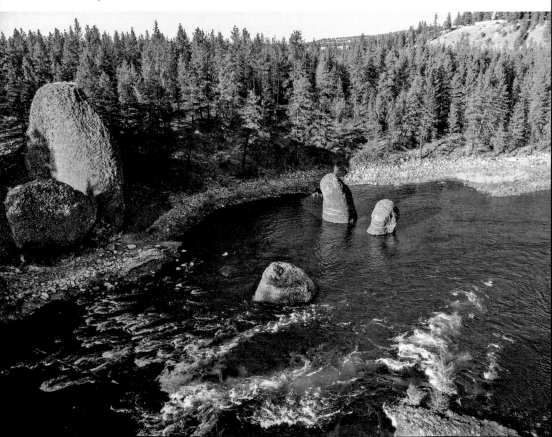

# KEY INFORMATION

**CONTACT:** 509-465-5064, state.wa.us/573/Riverside

**OPEN:** Year-round (Bowl and Pitcher, Equestrian subject to closure during heavy snowfall); April 15–October 31 (Nine Mile Recreation Area, Lake Spokane)

**SITES:** 103 across 4 campgrounds (Bowl and Pitcher: 34 total—16 standard, 16 with electricity and water, 2 group [one for 20–60 people, one for 20–40 people]; Equestrian: 21 total—10 equestrian with corrals, 11 with electricity, 10 with no hookups; Nine Mile: 24 total—3 tent sites, 21 full hookup; Lake Spokane: about 23 total—11 primitive sites and 4 boat-in areas with about 1–3 sites each)

**EACH SITE HAS:** Picnic table, fire pit with grill

**ASSIGNMENT:** First come, first served, or by reservation at 888-CAMPOUT (888-226-7688) or washington.goingtocamp.com

**REGISTRATION:** On-site, online, or by phone

**AMENITIES:** Bowl and Pitcher: Dump station, 2 restrooms (both with showers); Equestrian: 2 restrooms, water, arena, several hundred acres with loop trails and 40 miles of linear trails for horseback riding; Nine Mile: Swimming area, boat launch, 3 kitchen shelters with water and electricity (2 can hold up to 40 people, 1 holds up to 20 people), interpretive center; Lake Spokane: Vault toilet, no water or electricity, no garbage service

**PARKING:** At individual sites

**FEE:** $20–$35 standard, $25–$45 with partial to full utilities, $12 primitive

**ELEVATION:** 1,702'

---

**RESTRICTIONS:**

**PETS:** On leash only

**FIRES:** In fire pits only

**ALCOHOL:** Permitted

**VEHICLES:** Trailers and RVs up to 45' at Bowl and Pitcher (limited number available)

or kayaking. Whether you live near Spokane or are coming into town for a concert, to visit friends and family, or to bask in the natural beauty of the area—of Riverside State Park itself or nearby Mount Spokane or Coeur D'Alene, Idaho—the park is a wonderful option for camping. It's close to the city center if you want to go out to eat, shop, or attend a literary reading, but if you bring all your supplies, you don't have to leave.

**Bowl and Pitcher** is one of the most popular areas—not just for camping but for day use. Its name comes from the rock formation in the river, not too far from its 34 campsites (16 standard, 16 with full utility hookups, and 2 large group campsites for up to 60 people). This area is a great launch point for hiking, trail running, or general meandering. It's very close to the suspension bridge, which was built by the Civilian Conservation Corps. Cross the bridge from the campground and day-use area and—poof—you're in nature. You can go in any direction you like. You'll see ponderosa pines, basalt formations, rocky outcroppings and bluffs, and—of course—the river. The 2-mile loop trail is a popular walk to get a feel for the place. But remember that there are miles and miles of trails to explore on foot, on bicycle, and on horseback—about 80 miles' worth in the entire park.

The **Equestrian Campground** (and you don't have to have a horse to camp there), is located just south of Bowl and Pitcher, on the other side of the Spokane River. If you do bring your horse, there's a 60-foot pen, a 140-by-240-foot arena, a trail course with obstacles, and 21 campsites (10 with corrals, 11 with electricity). If Bowl and Pitcher is full, it's worth checking here because the campsites are extra spacious and there may be fewer people than other areas of the park. It's pricey but each site can accommodate up to eight people and three tents. Plus, you might get to make friends with a horse.

**Nine Mile Recreation Area** has 24 sites, 21 ideal for RVs and 3 for tent camping (a dump station and kitchen shelters with electricity are available), so in general I'd steer clear of this area for camping. The view of the river is beautiful, but leave it to the trailers. Though you should know that from May 15 to September 15 you can rent canoes and kayaks at Nine Mile, and there's a small park store with some basic supplies, as well as wood and ice. There are more trails here, including Indian Painted Rocks, as well as a boat launch. So don't avoid visiting this section of the park even if its campground isn't the best fit for you.

**Lake Spokane Campground,** also called Long Lake Campground, sits on a bluff above the lake. There's a beautiful panoramic view, and you have your pick of 11 primitive camp-sites. This is a choice spot. It's worth the drive up there to see if it's the right fit for you. Water access is a quick drive down to the base of the bluff, and there are options for swim-ming or boating from there, at the Lake Spokane boat launch.

Here's where it gets good: four first-come, first-served boat-in campsites are accessible from the Lake Spokane boat launch. Each site has a campfire ring with grate and picnic table, and there's a vault toilet. It feels very remote even though you're practically in Spo-kane. You can park at the Lake Spokane Campground or Nine Mile Recreation Area (dis-play your Discover Pass). If you have a boat or want to rent a canoe or kayak, you can make the trip and experience something really special. If there's no way you're going to boat to

Bowl and Pitcher suspension bridge

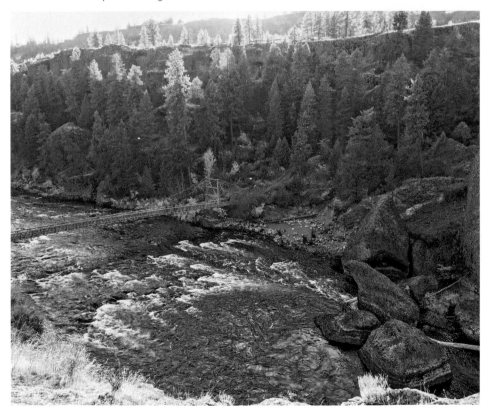

your campsite, I'd stick with the bluff or Bowl and Pitcher, depending on what you're in the mood for. The bluff will be a bit quieter, but it accommodates RVs. Bowl and Pitcher has RVs, but they're in their own area.

Once you're set up, explore! The Spokane River Centennial State Park Trail is nearly 40 miles of paved trail that goes all the way to Idaho. If you're ready to lace up your roller skates or hop on a bicycle, 13 miles of the trail run through Riverside State Park. No matter what time of year you make your trip, the extensive trails are sure to impress.

## GETTING THERE

From I-90, take Exit 280 and travel north across Maple Street Bridge. Turn left on West Maxwell Avenue, then continue onto North Pettet Drive. Take a slight left into the park entrance at Bowl and Pitcher.

**GPS COORDINATES** N47° 41.725' W117° 29.641'

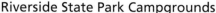

### Riverside State Park Campgrounds

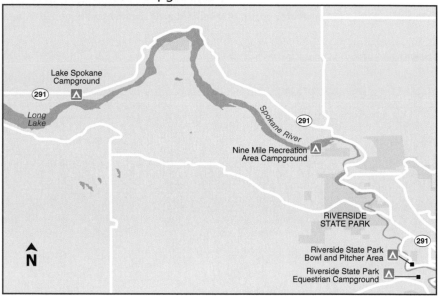

## Bowl and Pitcher Campground

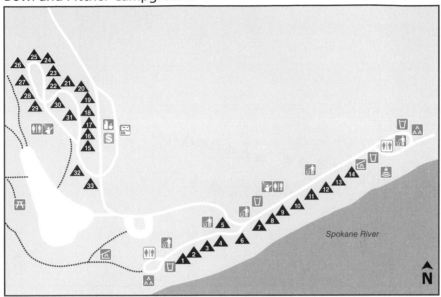

## Equestrian Campground

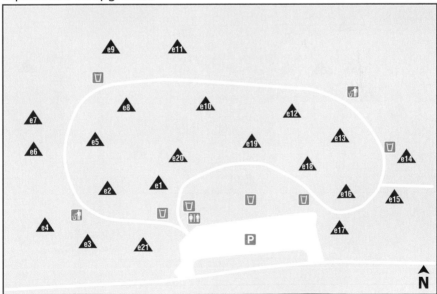

*See next page for Nine Mile Recreation Area and*
*Lake Spokane Campground maps.*

## Nine Mile Recreation Area Campground

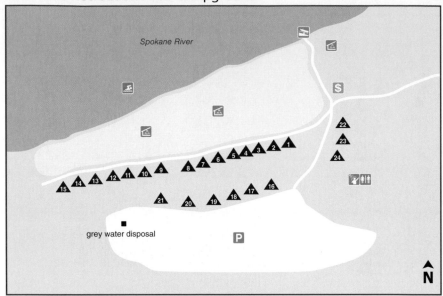

## Lake Spokane Campground

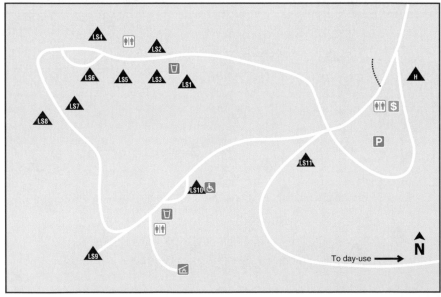

# SOUTHEASTERN WASHINGTON

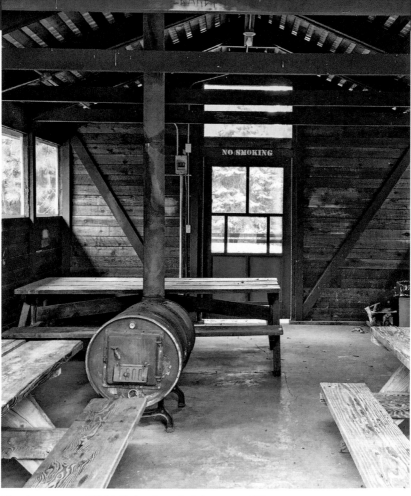

The day-use area at Fields Spring State Park (see page 169)

# 47

# Brooks Memorial State Park Campground

Beauty ★★★ Privacy ★★★ Spaciousness ★★★ Quiet ★★★★★ Security ★★★★ Cleanliness ★★★★★

*In the Simcoe Mountains, Brooks Memorial makes an excellent by-the-highway spot for exploring the lovely scenery of Klickitat Valley.*

In the early days of my short-lived career as a river-rafting guide, I was part of the historic first commercial descent of the Klickitat River, a small, lively, and rapidly dropping tumble of water that courses off the slopes of Gilbert Peak high in the Goat Rocks Wilderness. Plunging south through the basalt-lined canyons of the Yakama Indian Reservation east of Mount Adams, the Klickitat finally succumbs to anonymity as it empties into the Columbia River at the small town of Lyle.

It was my dubious luck to hang around with a ragtag group of egocentric boaters who were always seeking the aquatic version of "steep and deep." You skiers know what I mean.

The Klickitat fit the bill—steep and narrow descents, nightmarish S curves, and boulders and logs everywhere. To make a long story short, the river won. Klickitat, 2; humiliated ragtag group of boaters, 0.

Fortunately you'll find more than just hair-raising river running to keep you busy if you're in the Goldendale area and need a campground for the night. From its 3,000-foot location in the Simcoe Mountains, Brooks Memorial State Park is a good base for exploring not only the Klickitat Valley but also sights farther south toward the Columbia River, west into the untamed Klickitat River region and to Mount Adams, and north along the Yakama Indian Reservation and into the viticultural lands of the Yakima Valley.

Fall and spring are the best times to enjoy the park's 9 miles of hiking trails.

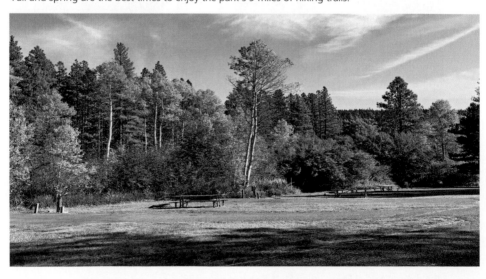

## KEY INFORMATION

**CONTACT:** 509-773-4611, Brooks Memorial State Park; 360-905-8544, Washington State Parks; parks.state.wa.us

**OPEN:** April 1–October 28

**SITES:** 22 standard, 23 with utilities

**EACH SITE HAS:** Picnic table, fire pit with grill

**ASSIGNMENT:** First come, first served, or by reservation at 888-CAMPOUT (888-226-7688) or washington.goingtocamp.com

**REGISTRATION:** Self-registration, online, by phone

**AMENITIES:** Restrooms with flush toilets, sinks, showers; 2 kitchen shelters with picnic tables, sinks, electricity; playground; group camp, horseshoe pits; potable water; hookups for RVs at some sites

**PARKING:** At campground and at individual sites

**FEE:** $20–$45 standard and utility, $12 primitive, $10 each additional vehicle

**ELEVATION:** 2,600'

---

**RESTRICTIONS:**

**PETS:** On leash only

**FIRES:** In fire pit only, wood gathering prohibited

**ALCOHOL:** Permitted at campsite or picnic site

**VEHICLES:** RVs up to 60' (limited site availability)

There are many points of interest in all directions. Central to the area is Goldendale, a quiet community that is home to the Goldendale Observatory State Park Interpretive Center and one of the largest telescopes open to the public in the country.

Down along the Columbia, historical attractions include Maryhill Museum and the American version of Stonehenge. Maryhill Museum houses the world-famous art collection of Sam—who-in-the-Sam-Hill—Hill and his wife, Mary. Also the brainchild of Hill, the Stonehenge Memorial, which copies its English namesake in size, honors Klickitat County's young men who fought and died in World War I.

The entire area around Goldendale had an eventful past. The Klickitat people have inhabited the region for hundreds of years and was instrumental in negotiating between eastern and western tribes who gathered in the region to trade and socialize. At Horse-Thief Lake State Park (on WA 14 along the Columbia), you can see Native American petroglyphs.

This is the dry side of the Cascades, which means hot and dry summers with cool nights. Winters are generally chilly and snowy. Brooks Memorial is open year-round and offers seasonal activities. Summer and fall are best for enjoying the 9 miles of hiking trails that follow the Little Klickitat River up into meadows for sensational up-close views of Mount Hood. Winter offers cross-country skiing, snowmobiling, and snowshoeing. Wildflowers bloom prolifically in the park from March until July, and there is quite a diversity of park wildlife at various times of the year: turkey, porcupine, beaver, bobcat, coyote, red-tailed hawk, and owl. The park even has a butterfly garden where 27 species have been sighted. The Little Klickitat River follows US 97 from Brooks Memorial down into Goldendale, and it's not uncommon to observe beavers going about their business of damming the river. Additional activities around Goldendale include golfing, windsurfing on the Columbia at Doug's Beach State Park, bicycling, and rock climbing.

Despite my tale of woe at the beginning of this chapter, river running is also an enjoyable option. Both the Klickitat and the White Salmon offer their share of thrills and chills. The characteristics of both rivers make them best suited to kayak descents, but our pioneering rafting effort has contributed to the popularity of rafting as well. Check out the local guide services for more information on this.

Your choice of campsite at Brooks Memorial will be based on what's available on their first-come, first-serve system. If it's a weekday, off-season, or winter, you'll get your pick of spacious sites. Go for the ones farthest from the road, which are, fortunately, tent sites 24–45 (although it's a lonely place, and at night cars are few). I noticed that some of the tent sites are a bit awkwardly positioned up the hillside, so finding a level spot for the tent can be a challenge. Foliage is thin between sites too, so finding privacy can also be a trial. The higher up the hillside you go, the more privacy and the more slope, so weigh your priorities accordingly.

## Brooks Memorial State Park Campground

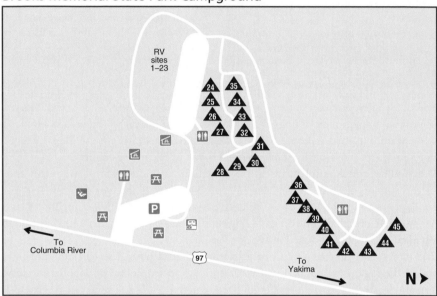

## GETTING THERE

From Yakima, follow US 97 south 55 miles, crossing Satus Pass (elevation 3,107') to the park entrance on the right. Administrative and maintenance buildings and the Environmental Learning Center are across US 97 on the left.

**GPS COORDINATES** N45° 56.926'  W120° 40.000'

# 48

# ⚠ Fields Spring State Park Campground

Beauty ★★★★ Privacy ★★★ Spaciousness ★★★★★ Quiet ★★★★ Security ★★★★ Cleanliness ★★★★★

*This park is a handy wilderness escape from Clarkston and Lewiston, an ideal layover between destinations north and south, or a destination of its own.*

Where the heck is Anatone? Even if you're a born-and-bred native Washingtonian, you may have to reach for the map on this one. I'll give you a hint. It's just south of Asotin. Need more clues? If you've ever traveled between Clarkston (Washington) and Enterprise (Oregon), you've driven right through Anatone. It's where you yawned and rubbed your eyes to stay awake.

Needless to say, Anatone is quite small—but it's significant in the world of tent camping. It's the last stop for any kind of services before one continues on to Fields Spring State Park. That means that anything you need that they didn't have in Anatone is all the way back in Clarkston or Lewiston (Idaho). Beyond Fields Spring to the south lies wilderness, national forest, and wild river canyons. Maybe you'd better make one last review of that checklist.

Literally on the edge of nowhere (which is where most tent campers like to find themselves), Fields Spring State Park is actually a handy wilderness escape for folks from Clarkston and Lewiston (both about 20 miles away). For anyone else, the park is an ideal layover between destinations north and south or can be a destination of its own. From Spokane, it's only two and a half hours. From the urban centers of western Washington and Oregon, it's easily an eight-hour drive. Admittedly, it's well off the beaten path, but that's part of its appeal. Besides, the roads are good all the way there. When the next long holiday weekend comes up, here's one to consider.

Sitting on a basalt foundation at 4,000 feet elevation on the eastern edge of Washington's Blue Mountains, Fields Spring State Park is open all year and hosts activities in every season. It's a place of unusual beauty in an otherwise harsh and rugged terrain, created by one of the largest and deepest lava flows in the world's geologic history. Evidence of this massive, recurring lava activity,

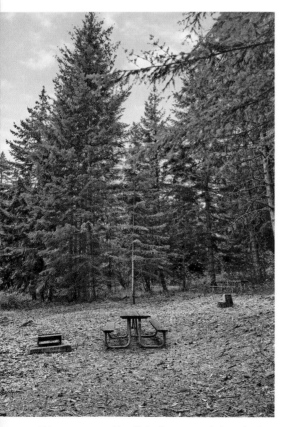

This campground is off the beaten path, but that's part of its appeal.

# KEY INFORMATION

**CONTACT:** 509-256-3332, Fields Spring State Park; 360-905-8544, Washington State Parks; parks.state.wa.us

**OPEN:** Year-round, snow park permit needed November 15–April 30

**SITES:** 20 standard

**EACH SITE HAS:** Picnic table, fire pit with grill, shade trees

**ASSIGNMENT:** First come, first served, or by reservation at 888-CAMPOUT (888-226-7688) or washington.goingtocamp.com

**REGISTRATION:** Self-registration on-site, online, by phone

**AMENITIES:** Bathhouse with sinks, toilets, showers, hot water; kitchen shelter with electricity; woodstove; firewood; public telephone; playground; environmental learning center with 2 lodges for group rental; restaurant and ice nearby; dump station

**PARKING:** At individual sites

**FEE:** $20–$35 standard, $12 primitive

**ELEVATION:** 4,000'

---

**RESTRICTIONS:**

**PETS:** On leash only

**FIRES:** In fire pit only

**ALCOHOL:** Permitted

**VEHICLES:** Trailers and RVs up to 30'

known as the Columbia Plateau, can best be seen in the walls of river gorges and canyons throughout southeastern Washington.

One of the best places to view the canyons themselves is right at the state park. Unless you've brought your hang glider or parasail (an increasingly popular way to tour the area), a 1-mile hike up 4,500-foot Puffer Butte (elevation gain 500') provides vistas into both the Grande Ronde River and the mighty Snake River canyons and across Washington, Oregon, and Idaho, whose borders converge in this corner. While the Snake River is practically a household name, with its immensely popular boating adventures, the Grande Ronde is relatively obscure, wandering northeast from Oregon's Anthony Lakes region (see *Best Tent Camping: Oregon* if you're continuing on in that direction). Of its total 185 miles, the Washington stretch of the Grande Ronde is mostly a drift trip with Class II and III rapids. It's not considered a highly technical river, but deceptively powerful eddies during high water and rocks at low periods require you to be experienced.

Paddlers looking for greater technical challenges should venture upstream into the Oregon sector. Parts of the river's Oregon flow are designated wild and scenic, and there are several put-in spots not far from Fields Spring. Take a good road map of the area if you plan to do any shuttling.

Escaping the heat of the summer is one of the biggest draws to Fields Spring. Although the 792 park acres sit on what is essentially an arid, desertlike plateau with prickly pear cactus growing down along the Grande Ronde's banks, the difference in elevation makes all the difference in temperature. While Clarkston and Lewiston swelter in 100°F agony in midsummer, Fields Spring rarely gets above a tolerable 85°F. Hear that, Spokanites?

However, winter is a different story. Snowy conditions make for ideal cross-country ski outings, and the park staff maintains approximately 8 miles of trails.

In springtime, catch the spectacular wildflower display or see if you can identify all eight species of woodpeckers that nest in and among the stands of western larch, grand fir, Douglas-fir, and ponderosa pine shading the campsites.

The campground itself is a simple affair with 20 tent spaces that double as RV sites without hookups. There is no bad spot among the 20 unless you've got an inconsiderate neighbor. For a state park this small, it's indeed a treat to have restrooms with showers, so take advantage.

Whether you're passing through or making this corner of Washington the destination, Fields Spring is a true tent camper's oasis in a region otherwise parched for camping options.

## Fields Spring State Park

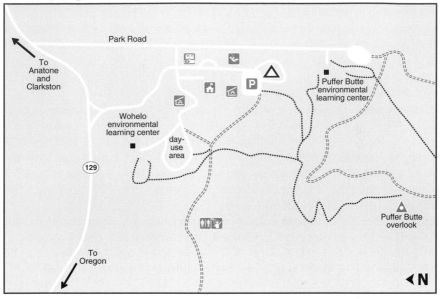

## GETTING THERE

From Clarkston (roughly 110 miles south of Spokane), follow WA 129 south through Asotin 21 miles and then head 4 miles past Anatone to the park entrance.

**GPS COORDINATES** N46° 05.210'  W117° 10.157'

# 49

# ⚠ Godman Campground

Beauty ★★★★ Privacy ★★★ Spaciousness ★★★★★ Quiet ★★★★★ Security ★★★ Cleanliness ★★★★★

*Perhaps named when Lewis said to Clark, "God, man, where in blazes are we?"*

For those of you looking for an ends-of-the-earth destination complete with (gulp!) stories of stalking mountain lions, read on. For those of you who prefer to find your own adventures rather than have them find you, try Fields Spring State Park.

Godman Campground is the sacred domain of modern-day explorers who have a healthy appetite for bone-jarring roads and cliff-hanging vistas, and an unflappable self-confidence in the face of some really badly marked U.S. Forest Service roads (or maybe it was just my map). At any rate, I think it's highly probable that even the intrepid Lewis and Clark found themselves scratching their heads up here.

Presto! A campground name was born!

If Tucannon, at a mere 2,600-foot elevation, is the last bastion of civilized camping adventure in the Umatilla, then Godman—at 6,050 feet—is the start of all things wild . . . beginning with stories we heard from a couple cruising through as part of an anniversary-weekend celebration. OK, that's not the wild part! Calamity Jane meets Davy Crockett, you may think. Actually, they couldn't have looked more suburban in their minivan and gawky white tennis shoes. Suddenly, I didn't feel very remote.

Turns out they had it on good authority that the mountain lion threat around Godman can be very real. We all shot quick glances around as we stood very obviously in the wide-open spaces of the U.S. Forest Service road, one eye on the tree limbs above. We talked louder than we needed to. We laughed nervously. Suddenly, I felt remote as hell.

This wilderness campground provides a splendid outback experience.

photographed by *Elizabeth A. Escher*

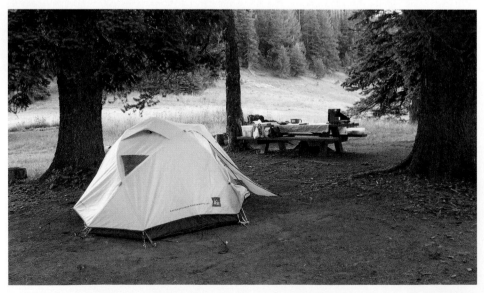

## KEY INFORMATION

**CONTACT:** 509-843-1891, tinyurl.com
/godmancampground

**OPEN:** Camping mid-June–late October,
weather permitting; cabin available all year

**SITES:** 8

**EACH SITE HAS:** Picnic table, fire pit with grill

**ASSIGNMENT:** First come, first served; cabin
rental and lookout reservations accepted at
recreation.gov or 877-444-6777

**REGISTRATION:** Not necessary for camping;
online or by phone for glamping

**AMENITIES:** Vault toilets; nonpotable water
for humans; hitching rails, feed troughs,
and spring for horses; group picnic shelter;
rentable guard station; no garbage service

**PARKING:** At individual sites

**FEE:** None

**ELEVATION:** 6,050'

---

**RESTRICTIONS:**

**PETS:** On leash only

**FIRES:** In fire pits only

**ALCOHOL:** Permitted

**VEHICLES:** RVs and trailers not
recommended

Well, as the Umatilla Forest Service advises you on its website, spending time in the wilderness involves an "element of risk." This caveat aside, Wenaha-Tucannon Wilderness is too splendid of an outback experience to let a few 250-pound cougars ruin it. However, it's worth checking with the ranger station before you go to see if there have been any incidents. Maybe that nice-looking couple in their ready-for-action tennis shoes have the right idea.

The campground at Godman is a terribly uncomplicated affair and very nearly unrecognizable as a campground unless you get out of the car and walk around. There are eight sites—so they say—and if this place were ever full, I would be very surprised! The most obvious sites are wrapped around the side of the heavily wooded ridge where FS 46 turns west into deep, dark unknowns and leaves the campground in a matter of seconds. A couple of sites are tucked back along a brushy spur road of sorts, but that looked like cougar-snoozing territory to me, so I wimped out on investigating further. You go first.

In the clearing below the road, the Godman Guard Station is a surprising discovery, even though I knew about it before I visited the campground. Built in the feverish 1930s by the Civilian Conservation Corps (those guys were everywhere!), the cabin is not doing much guarding these days but is fully furnished and available for rent year-round (although winter requires that one have the fortitude of the Nez Perce, whose numbers were once great, to get in here via skis, snowshoes, or snowmobile). Even more surprising, the cabin didn't appear to be rented at the height of the summer season, so it seems reasonable to imagine snagging it when you want.

Fortunately, whoever found this elbow in the road and claimed it for the Umatilla National Forest made sure that the main attractions—views to the south and west—were visible from every campsite. From this high ridge literally at the western door of Wenaha-Tucannon Wilderness, gorgeous sunsets are the evening entertainment while you're cooking dinner.

Daytime entertainment is also right at your fingertips. The 200-mile network of trails in Wenaha-Tucannon can be accessed from West Butte Creek Trail 3138. You could conceivably wander for days and not see another living (two-footed) soul. You'll wear yourself out in the process. Most of the trails in Wenaha-Tucannon make steep, abrupt drops into the river and creek canyons, only to climb back up through thick forests of fir, spruce, pine, hemlock, and western larch to the expansive plateaus. It's a roller-coaster ride through Wenaha-Tucannon.

If you want to start high and stay high, the best route is the ridgetop run 3113—known as Mount Misery Trail. It connects Teepee Trailhead (just below Godman at 5,400') and Diamond Trail, which leaves from the base of Diamond Peak, the second-highest point in the wilderness at 6,379 feet. The Diamond Trail goes on to skirt Oregon Butte, the wilderness's high point at 6,401 feet with a side trip to a lookout with jaw-dropping, 360-degree views!

## Godman Campground

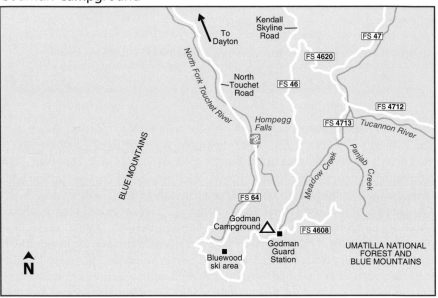

## GETTING THERE

From Dayton, turn right on CR 118, which starts as Eckler Mountain Road and becomes Skyline Drive. Travel 14 miles to FS 46 (a continuation of Skyline Drive) and follow it 11 miles to the campground. Have very good county and U.S. Forest Service maps with you both to find Godman and to more deeply explore the labyrinth of roads in lower Columbia County.

**GPS COORDINATES**  N46° 06.050'  W117° 47.142'

# 50

# ⚠ Palouse Falls State Park Campground

Beauty ★★★★ Privacy ★ Spaciousness ★★★★ Quiet ★★★★★ Security ★★ Cleanliness ★★★★★

*With a spectacular waterfall in the middle of the eastern Washington steppes, this is a fantastic spot for camping—if you can manage to have it to yourself.*

On a stinking hot summer morning (in Bellingham), I packed up the car, picked up a friend, and made a beeline for the remote reaches of Washington's famous grasslands. And I have to say that, despite the minimal offerings at Palouse Falls, there are certain redeeming tent-camping qualities about the park that make it imperative for me to fly directly in the face of those who say it's worthless and go ahead and recommend it to all of you.

First, no one in their right mind would imagine camping there, so you'll have the place to yourself by sundown (at least the camping area), right? Right?

Palouse Falls drops 200 feet into the canyon below.

photographed by *Lisa Laughlin*

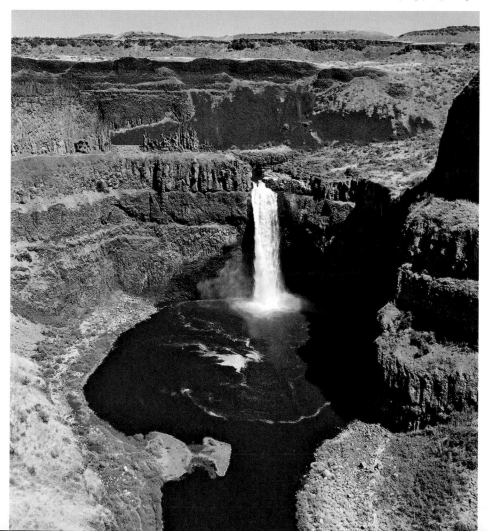

**CONTACT:** 509-646-9218, Palouse Falls State Park; 360-905-8544, Washington State Parks; parks.state.wa.us

**OPEN:** Year-round

**SITES:** 11 tent-only

**EACH SITE HAS:** Picnic table, fire pit, raised brazier

**ASSIGNMENT:** First come, first served

**REGISTRATION:** On-site

**AMENITIES:** Vault toilets, no water in winter, picnic area, dump station

**PARKING:** In general parking area

**FEE:** $12, $10 each additional vehicle

**ELEVATION:** 750'

**RESTRICTIONS:**

**PETS:** On leash only

**FIRES:** In fire pit only

**ALCOHOL:** Permitted

**VEHICLES:** No RV or pickup-and-camper parking

---

Second, this is a world away from anything that Westsiders experience on a daily basis and just from sheer novelty gets my vote. Desert. Canyon. Waterfall. The Palouse!

Third, the place is too full of geological and archaeological significance to imagine that the parks department would close this facility. And the more people use it, the less likely it will be to close. They've already been forced to do that with Lyons Ferry, Central Ferry, and Chief Timothy State Parks. A disturbing trend, to be sure.

Fourth, in light of point three, there aren't nearly the camping options in this region that there were even as recently as a year ago, so from a tent-camping standpoint, Palouse Falls is a winner. Perhaps the long-term plan, given the closure of the much larger neighboring facilities, is to make improvements to Palouse Falls. One can only hope.

On that note, I should prepare you in advance for what you'll find: very little in the way of campground amenities. But much in the way of atmosphere, adventure, and austerity.

The camping area is nothing more than an open, grassy patch with a few spindly shade trees up to the left as you drive in. Yup, that's it. Raised brazier grills are positioned in an attempt to define individual sites, but for the most part, spacing will be determined by how much each camping party is willing to concede. If you're inclined toward sprawl, the spaces are going to get small in a hurry.

Let's put it in perspective. The entire park sits on 105 acres, and that includes a fair bit of land that is mostly undeveloped and through which trails wind along the canyon rim to various overlooks for viewing the falls. The camping area is part of only 2 acres that includes the picnicking area as well. The parking lot is bigger than the campground, if that helps give you a visual. Whatever you do, don't rely on the state park website to give you a picture of camping at Palouse Falls. It's not so much what they say about the place; it's what they don't say. Based on their information, you would be tempted to come here expecting to find more of, well, a campground.

I hope you realize that this information is not meant to deter you. I just think it's important for you to know the score so there are no recriminations later. If the utmost in simplified camping is your style, then Palouse Falls will tickle you to no end.

Since the main attraction isn't the campground anyway, let's focus on what is: Palouse Falls, best visited in spring and early summer when the Palouse River dumps tons of water carrying tons of rich Palouse topsoil over the edge. It's a staggering scene but not exactly a pretty picture, with volumes of water about the color of a tall Starbucks double mocha with plenty of extra foam roaring into a 200-foot chasm. Later in the season, the flow becomes much clearer and also much quieter, enhancing the scale of the tortured basalt walls that form the deep amphitheater. Every year it seems someone or other gets stranded (or reaches their fatal end) attempting to hike down to the pool at the bottom. Do not do this. There is some hiking nearby, but this is steep and dangerous. Rangers are often posted here to warn you, but I'm warning you as well. Go hike around the area and dip your legs into the pools of water in the heat of summer—and enjoy the falls and their basalt walls from a safe viewpoint.

There's an Native American legend about those walls. Interpretive signs around the canyon perimeter tell of the creation of Palouse Falls and its singular importance as the vestige of a dramatic geologic event 15,000 years ago. If you want to read an excellent technical account of the shaping of this natural wonder, get a copy of *Hiking Washington's Geology (The Mountaineers)*—a good book to keep in the glove compartment (right beside this guide).

Just as fascinating as the falls is the Marmes Rock Shelter, where human remains have been dated as some of the oldest (roughly 10,000 years) found in the Western Hemisphere. You can access this site from the (former) Lyons Ferry Park and Marina parking lot.

## Palouse Falls State Park Campground

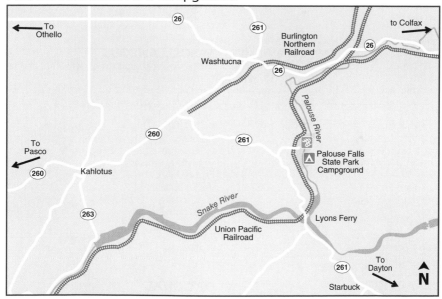

## GETTING THERE

From Washtucna at the intersection of WA 26 and WA 261, travel about 6 miles south on WA 261 to the junction of WA 260. Turn left (southeast) onto WA 261 and drive 14.5 miles to Palouse Falls Road. Turn left and follow it less than 2 miles to the park.

**GPS COORDINATES** N46° 39.808′ W118° 13.657′

# APPENDIX A

# CAMPING EQUIPMENT CHECKLIST

Except for the large and bulky items on this list, I keep a plastic storage container full of the essentials for car camping so they're ready to go when I am. I make a last minute check of the inventory, resupply anything that's low or missing, and away I go!

## COOKING UTENSILS

Aluminum foil
Bear canister
Bottle opener
Can opener
Condiments *(salt, pepper, spices, sugar, cooking oil, maple syrup)* in waterproof, spill-proof containers
Corkscrew
Cups *(plastic or tin)*
Dish soap *(biodegradable)*, sponge, and towel
Flatware
Food of your choice
Frying pan
Fuel for stove
Matches in waterproof container
Plates
Pocketknife
Pot with lid
Potholder
Spatula
Stove
Water filter/tablets
Wooden spoon

## FIRST AID KIT

Band-Aids
First aid cream
Gauze pads
Ibuprofen or aspirin
Insect repellent
Moleskin
Snakebite kit *(if you're heading for desert conditions)*
Sunscreen, lip balm
Tape, waterproof adhesive

## SLEEPING GEAR

Pillow
Sleeping bag
Sleeping pad *(inflatable or insulated)*
Tent with ground tarp and rainfly

## MISCELLANEOUS

Bath soap *(biodegradable)*, washcloth, and towel
Camp chair
Candles
Cooler
Deck of cards
Fire starter
Flashlight with fresh batteries
Inclement-weather clothing *(useful year-round in the Northwest)*
Paper towels
Plastic ziplock bags
Sunglasses
Toilet paper
Trowel
Water bottle
Wet wipes
Wool blanket

## OPTIONAL

Barbecue grill
Bear spray
Binoculars
Books on bird, plant, and wildlife identification
Firewood *(buy near your campground)*
Fishing rod and tackle
Hammock
Hatchet
Lantern
Maps *(road, topographic, trails)*

# APPENDIX B

# SOURCES OF INFORMATION

## AAA AUTOMOBILE CLUB OF WASHINGTON
1523 15th Ave. W.
Seattle, WA 98119
206-218-1222
aaa.com

## CASCADE BICYCLE CLUB
7787 62nd Ave. NE
Seattle, WA 98115
206-522-3222 or 206-522-BIKE (2453)
*(ride-description hotline)*
cascade.org

## DISCOVER YOUR NORTHWEST
*(nonprofit information service)*
164 S. Jackson St.
Seattle, WA 98104
206-382-4232
discovernw.org

## LAKE ROOSEVELT NATIONAL RECREATION AREA
**(National Park Service)**
1008 Crest Drive
Coulee Dam, WA 99116
509-754-7800
nps.gov/laro

## MOUNT RAINIER NATIONAL PARK
**(National Park Service)**
Tahoma Woods, Star Route
55210 238th Ave. E.
Ashford, WA 98304
360-569-2211
nps.gov/mora

## MOUNT ST. HELENS NATIONAL VOLCANIC MONUMENT
**(U.S. Forest Service)**
42218 NE Yale Bridge Road
Amboy, WA 98601
360-449-7800
fs.fed.us/giffordpinchot

## THE MOUNTAINEERS
*(hiking and climbing club)*
7700 Sand Point Way NE
Seattle, WA 98115
206-521-6000
mountaineers.org

## NATIONAL RECREATION RESERVATION SYSTEM
877-444-6777
recreation.gov

## NORTH CASCADES NATIONAL PARK **(National Park Service)**
810 WA 20
Sedro-Woolley, WA 98284
360-854-7200
nps.gov/noca

## OLYMPIC NATIONAL PARK
**(National Park Service)**
600 E. Park Ave.
Port Angeles, WA 98362
360-565-3130
nps.gov/olym

## THE RANGER STATION AT REI
*(a partnership of the National Park Service, U.S. Forest Service, Washington State Parks, and REI)*
222 Yale North (inside REI)
Seattle, WA 98109-5429
800-270-7504 or 206-470-4060

## U.S. FOREST SERVICE
**(Pacific Northwest Regional Headquarters)**
P.O. Box 3623, Portland, OR 97208
333 SW First Ave., Portland, OR 97208
503-808-2468
fs.fed.us/r6

## WASHINGTON KAYAK CLUB
P.O. Box 98086
Lakewood, WA 98496
washingtonkayakclub.org

# SOURCES OF INFORMATION *(continued)*

**WASHINGTON STATE DEPT. OF COMMERCE AND ECONOMIC DEVELOPMENT, TOURISM DIVISION**
800-544-1800
experiencewa.com

**WASHINGTON STATE DEPT. OF FISH AND WILDLIFE**
Natural Resources Building
1111 Washington St. SE
Olympia, WA 98501
360-902-2200
wdfw.wa.gov

**WASHINGTON STATE DEPT. OF NATURAL RESOURCES**
P.O. Box 47000
1111 Washington St. SE
Olympia, WA 98504-7000
360-902-1000
dnr.wa.gov

**WASHINGTON STATE PARKS AND RECREATION COMMISSION**
P.O. Box 42650
Olympia, WA 98504
360-902-8844
parks.wa.gov

**WASHINGTON TRAILS ASSOCIATION**
705 Second Ave., Ste. 300
Seattle, WA 98104
206-625-1367
wta.org

**WASHINGTON WATER TRAILS ASSOCIATION**
4649 Sunnyside Ave. N., #307
Seattle, WA 98103
206-545-9161
wwta.org

# INDEX

# ABOUT THE AUTHORS

**Ellie Kozlowski** grew up in a suburb of Boston and camped on Cape Cod as a kid. She's lived in the Pacific Northwest for the better part of a decade. It is, she thinks, the best place to enjoy the desert, the rainforest, the ocean, and the mountains. She loves adventuring, hiking, stargazing, snowshoeing, reading or napping in her hammock, and losing cell service. When she's not driving up a mountainside or along a coast, she's enjoying all Seattle has to offer with her partner and their dog.

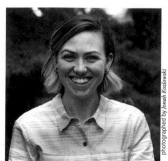

*photographed by Jonah Kozlowski*

**Jeanne Louise Pyle** lived in the Pacific Northwest for 30 years. Her love of the outdoors led to authoring the first book of the *Best Tent Camping* series in 1994.

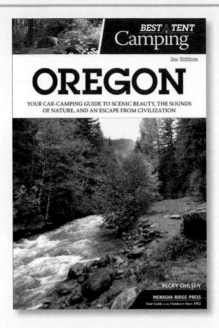

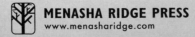

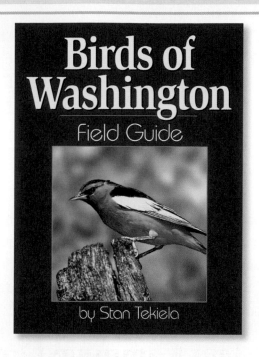

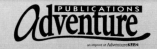

**DEAR CUSTOMERS AND FRIENDS,**

**SUPPORTING YOUR INTEREST IN OUTDOOR ADVENTURE,** travel, and an active lifestyle is central to our operations, from the authors we choose to the locations we detail to the way we design our books. Menasha Ridge Press was incorporated in 1982 by a group of veteran outdoorsmen and professional outfitters. For many years now, we've specialized in creating books that benefit the outdoors enthusiast.

Almost immediately, Menasha Ridge Press earned a reputation for revolutionizing outdoors- and travel-guidebook publishing. For such activities as canoeing, kayaking, hiking, backpacking, and mountain biking, we established new standards of quality that transformed the whole genre, resulting in outdoor-recreation guides of great sophistication and solid content. Menasha Ridge Press continues to be outdoor publishing's greatest innovator.

The folks at Menasha Ridge Press are as at home on a whitewater river or mountain trail as they are editing a manuscript. The books we build for you are the best they can be, because we're responding to your needs. Plus, we use and depend on them ourselves.

We look forward to seeing you on the river or the trail. If you'd like to contact us directly, visit us at menasharidge.com. We thank you for your interest in our books and the natural world around us all.

**SAFE TRAVELS,**

*Bob Sehlinger*

**BOB SEHLINGER**
**PUBLISHER**